HI-TECH HEALTH CARE

ROBOTICS IN HEALTH CARE

by Sue Bradford Edwards

BrightPoint Press

San Diego, CA

BrightPoint Press

© 2022 BrightPoint Press
an imprint of ReferencePoint Press, Inc.
Printed in the United States

For more information, contact:
BrightPoint Press
PO Box 27779
San Diego, CA 92198
www.BrightPointPress.com

ALL RIGHTS RESERVED.

No part of this work covered by the copyright hereon may be reproduced or used in any form or by any means—graphic, electronic, or mechanical, including photocopying, recording, taping, web distribution, or information storage retrieval systems—without the written permission of the publisher.

LIBRARY OF CONGRESS CATALOGING-IN-PUBLICATION DATA

Names: Edwards, Sue Bradford, author.
Title: Robotics in health care / by Sue Bradford Edwards.
Description: San Diego, CA : BrightPoint Press, [2022] | Series: Hi-tech health care | Includes bibliographical references and index. | Audience: Grades 7-9
Identifiers: LCCN 2021009948 (print) | LCCN 2021009949 (eBook) | ISBN 9781678201883 (hardback) | ISBN 9781678201890 (eBook)
Subjects: LCSH: Robotics in medicine--Juvenile literature. | Medical technology--Juvenile literature. | Robots--Juvenile literature.
Classification: LCC R857.R63 E39 2022 (print) | LCC R857.R63 (eBook) | DDC 610.285--dc23
LC record available at https://lccn.loc.gov/2021009948
LC eBook record available at https://lccn.loc.gov/2021009949

CONTENTS

AT A GLANCE	4
INTRODUCTION ROBOTIC SURGERY IN ACTION	6
CHAPTER ONE WHAT IS THE HISTORY OF ROBOTICS IN HEALTH CARE?	12
CHAPTER TWO HOW DO MEDICAL ROBOTS WORK?	24
CHAPTER THREE HOW ARE DOCTORS USING ROBOTS TODAY?	38
CHAPTER FOUR WHAT'S NEXT FOR ROBOTICS IN HEALTH CARE?	54
Glossary	74
Source Notes	75
For Further Research	76
Index	78
Image Credits	79
About the Author	80

AT A GLANCE

- A robot is a machine designed to do a job. A robot may do one job or many.

- The robot Unimate went to work in 1961. It was a robotic arm. It helped build cars for the company General Motors.

- Scientists at NASA were among the first to think about robots that could do surgery. Their goal was to help astronauts in space.

- Doctors commonly use robots in surgery today. Robots can reach where people cannot. They can make delicate, precise motions.

- Robots are used to deliver things in hospitals. They can carry meals or medicines. This frees up time for human hospital staff.

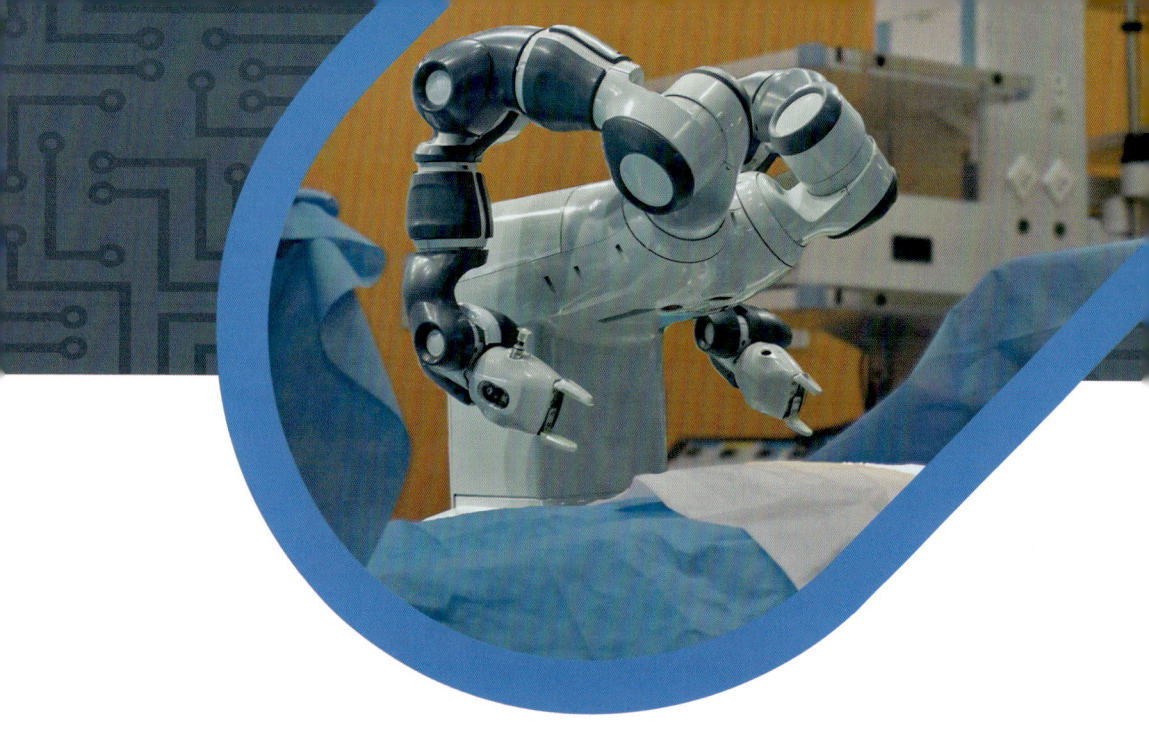

- Robots can help keep hospitals clean. They use ultraviolet light to kill germs.

- Some robots look like stuffed toys. They give patients comfort and help them heal.

- Robots can help people recover after an injury or illness. They can help someone learn to walk or regain strength.

- In the future, scientists may develop tiny robots that can work inside the human body.

INTRODUCTION

ROBOTIC SURGERY IN ACTION

A patient lies in the operating room. Beside him stands a robot. It has three thin arms. The end of one is a light. The end of another is a camera. The end of the third is a laser. The robot's arms reach into the patient's open mouth.

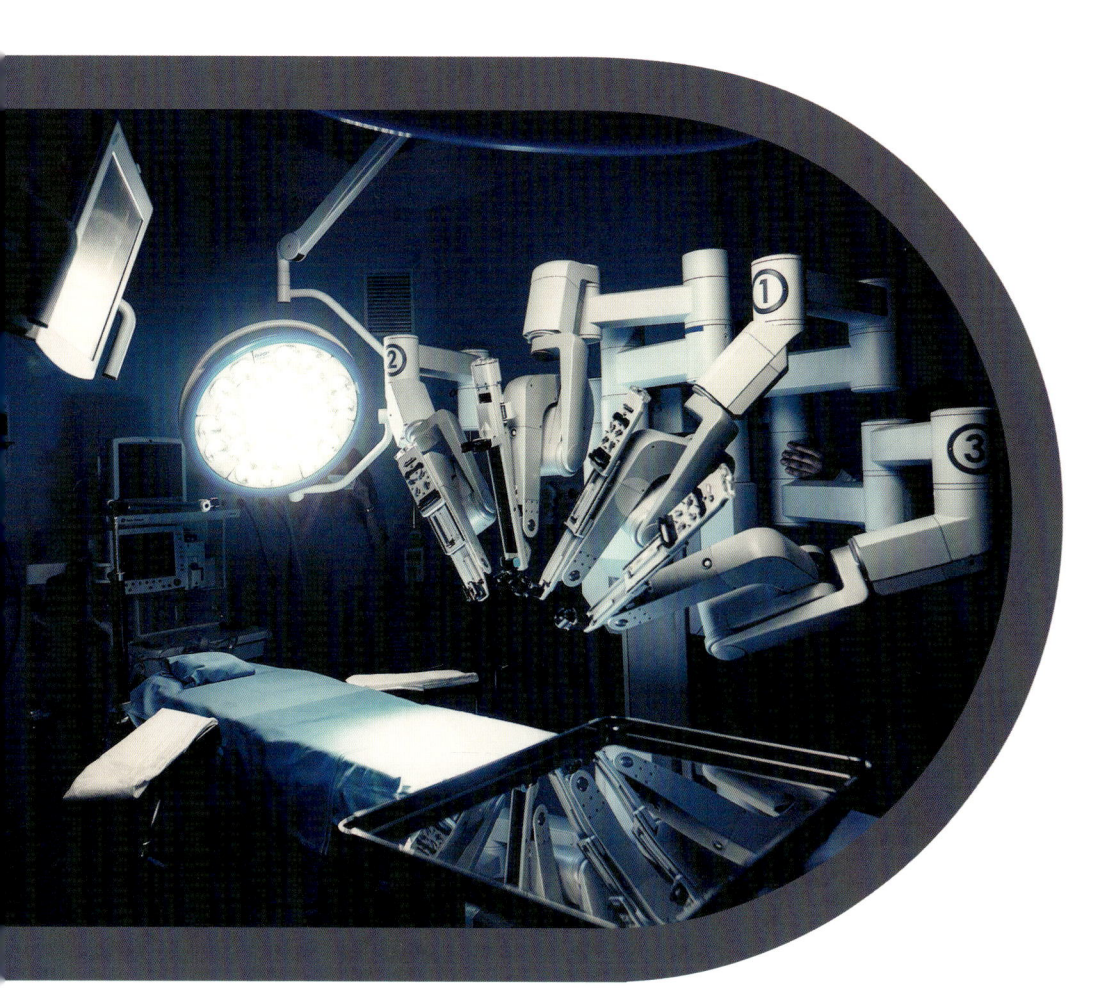

Medical robots sometimes have multiple arms with different abilities and features.

The patient has a tumor. It is in his throat. In the past, this tumor would be hard to reach. The surgeon might have had to

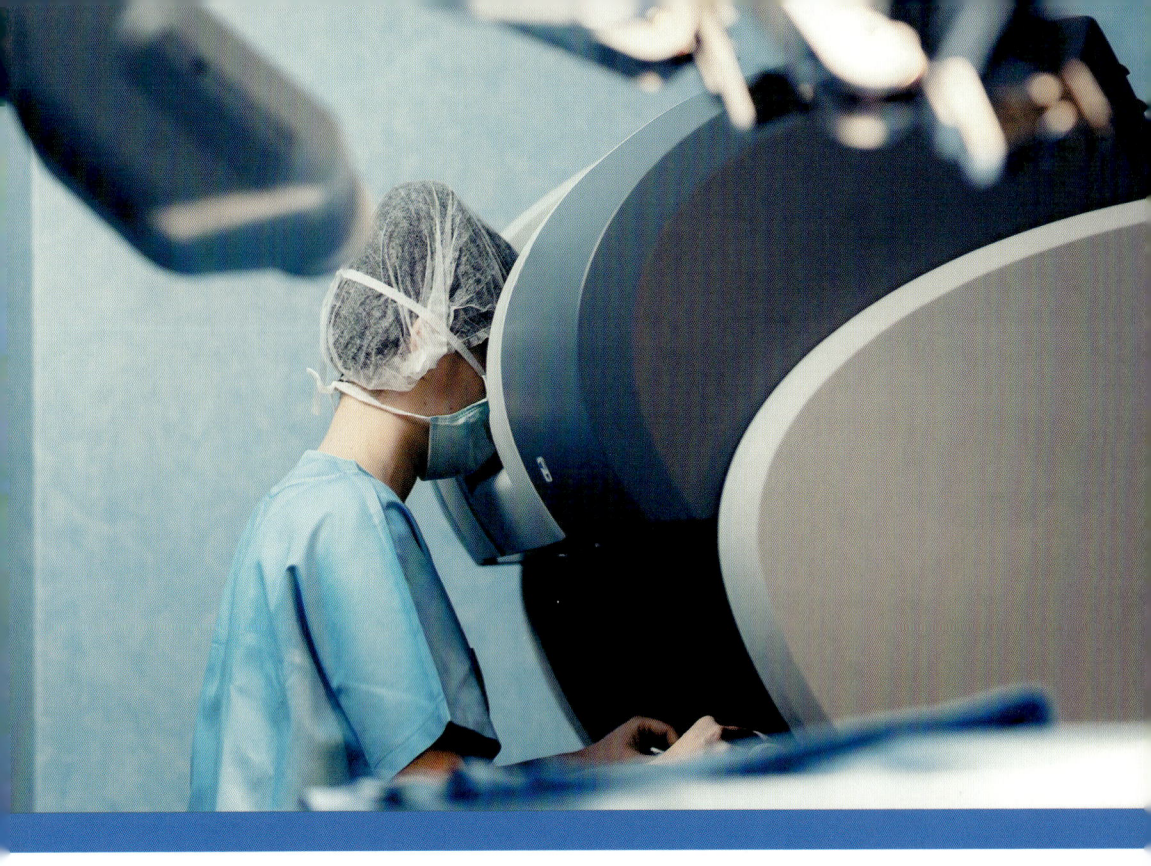

Doctors usually control surgery robots from a station nearby.

break the patient's jaw. She might have had to go in through his throat. But robot arms can bend. They can twist. They can reach the tumor.

The doctor sits nearby. She watches a screen. She sees what the camera sees.

She is looking at the tumor. Each of the doctor's hands is on a controller. She moves the robot's arms. She uses a laser to remove the tumor.

MEDICAL ROBOTS

A robot is a machine with a job to do. Doctors work with surgical robots. Some robots do one type of surgery. Some do several kinds. Other kinds of medical robots make deliveries in hospitals. Medical robots can also be used to kill germs.

To do these jobs, robots need tools. Some robots hold the tools. Sometimes the tools are built into the robot. Robots have

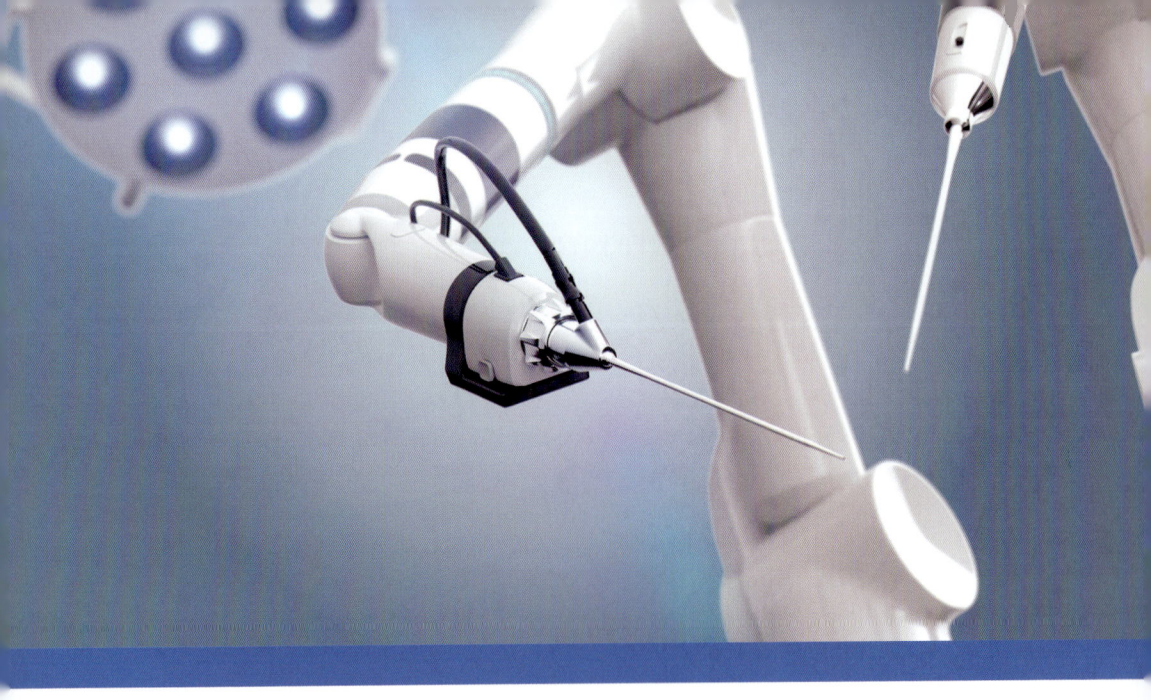

Surgery robots use a variety of tools.

lights and cameras. Some have lasers that can cut. Others have drills or saws.

Robots are controlled by computer programs. A program is a series of commands. The commands tell robots what to do and when to do it.

Unlike a person, a robot can work long hours without getting tired or bored. It can make small, exact movements. It can reach places that a person cannot. These traits make robots great assistants to human doctors.

Robots changed how doctors work. Removing a throat tumor used to take up to twelve hours. Now it takes ninety minutes. With no **incision**, the patient heals faster. "Patients that were in the hospital for . . . 14 days are now home the next day," says Dr. Eric M. Genden.[1] He is the director of the Head and Neck Cancer Center at Mt. Sinai Hospital in New York City. He has seen robots change patients' lives.

CHAPTER ONE

WHAT IS THE HISTORY OF ROBOTICS IN HEALTH CARE?

The first programmable robot was Unimate. In 1961, the car company General Motors used it in a factory. This robotic arm lifted hot metal. Scientists looked for other ways to use robots. Some people thought robots would make good

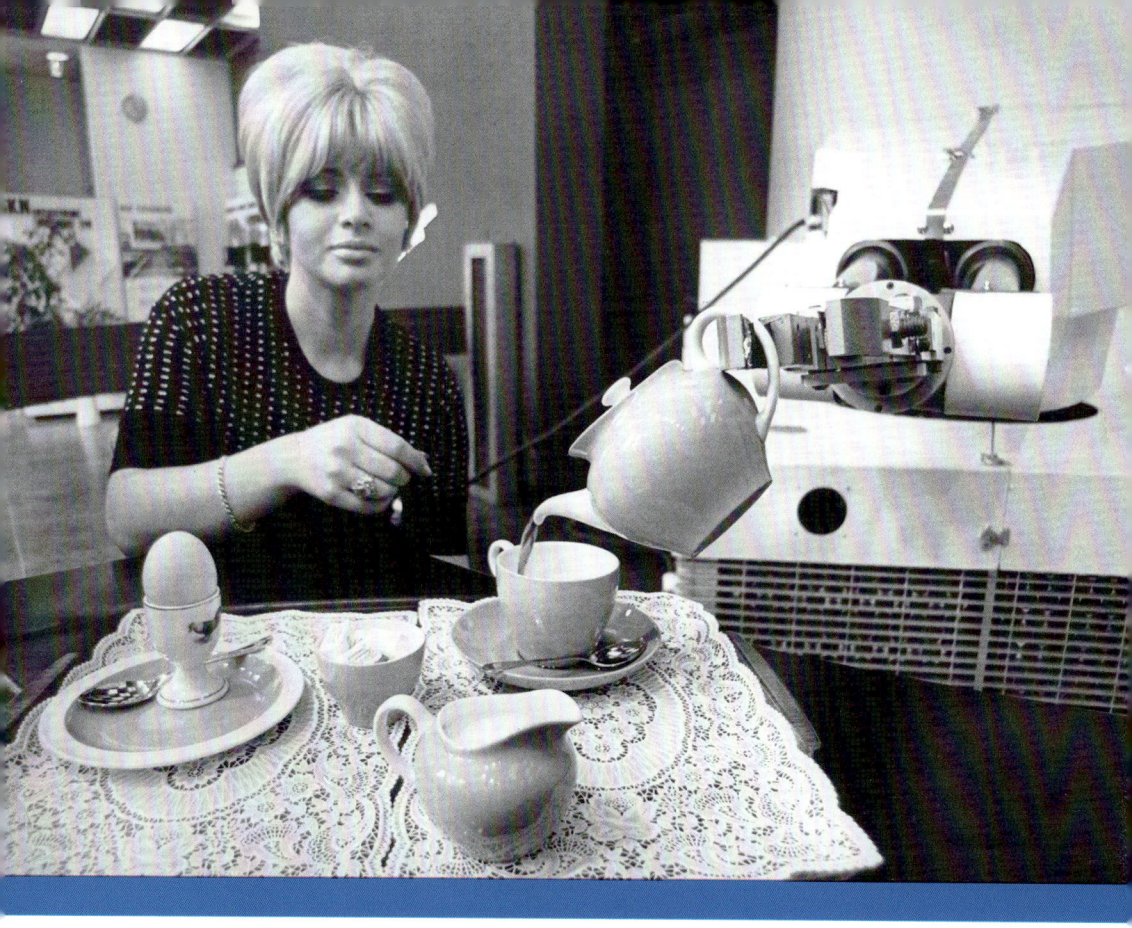

In a 1960s demonstration, a Unimate robot poured a cup of tea to show off its abilities.

teachers. They looked for ways robots could help young learners.

Other people looked for ways to use robots in space. In the 1970s, the National Aeronautics and Space Administration

(NASA) investigated this. NASA wanted to do tele-surgery. "Tele" means at a distance. The agency studied the idea of long-distance surgery. NASA worried an astronaut might get hurt or sick in space. NASA thought a doctor could work through

ROBOTS FOR CHILDREN

Robotic technology has been in toys for several decades. In 1978, parents could buy the Speak & Spell. It was built by Texas Instruments. It was a handheld computer. The computer would say a word. Then the child would type the word. By 1998, one robot toy looked like a stuffed animal. It was called Furby. When a person first bought one, Furby spoke Furbish. This was a language of nonsense words. Furby was programmed to use more English words over time.

a robot. The robot would be with the astronauts. The doctor would be on Earth. The doctor would direct the robot. However, scientists could not make it work. A signal takes time to travel a long distance. There is a delay before it reaches the other end. In surgery, this delay could be deadly.

    Surgery robots also had military uses. A soldier might need an operation in a war zone. A robotic arm could be in the dangerous area. A doctor could be someplace safe. He could remotely control the arm to operate.

SURGICAL ROBOTS

Scientists saw that robots could help operate. Robot arms can move in ways humans can't. They can make small, precise movements. This could make surgery faster, easier, and safer. Doctors and scientists got to work. They built many different robots.

ROBOT HELPERS

In the 1980s, the Stanford Robotic Aid Project opened. It was at Stanford University in California. Researchers built robot helpers. The robots would help injured soldiers. The robots would do more than one job. They could lift and move things. They could help users brush their teeth and shave. The robots would help people live on their own.

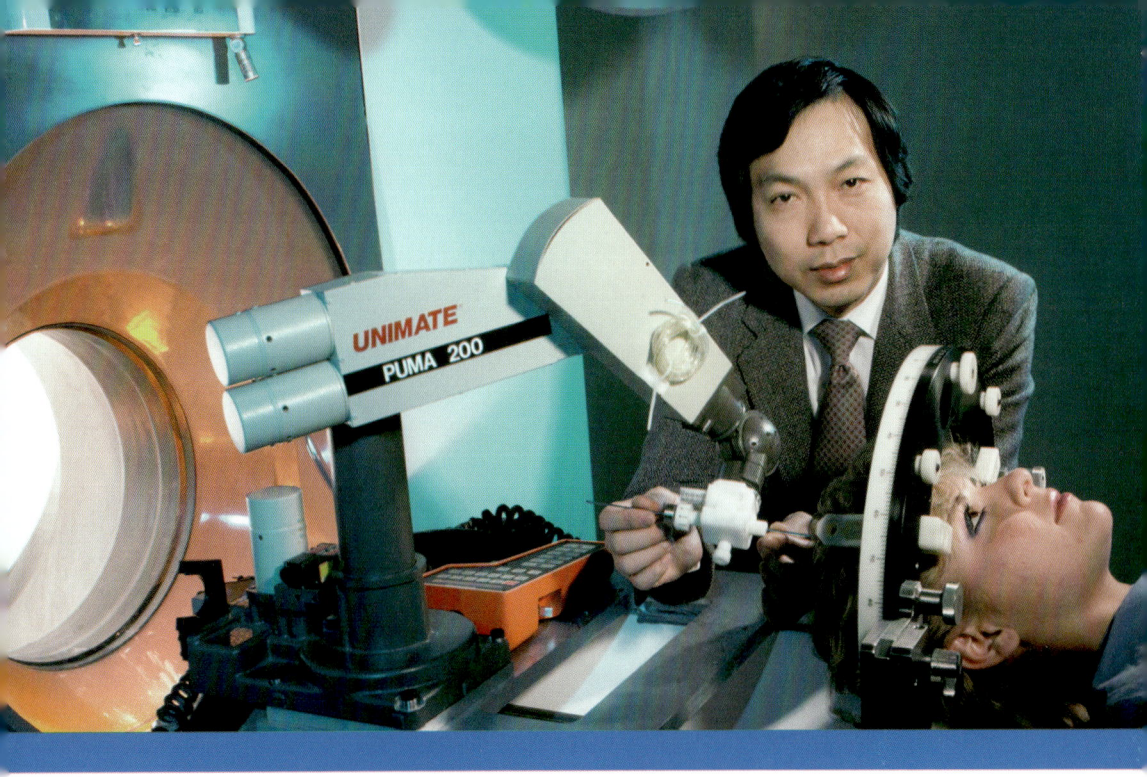

One of the creators of the PUMA 200, Dr. Yik San Kwoh, shows off the robot.

The PUMA 200 was the first surgical robot. A doctor first used it in 1985. First, he used a **CT scan** to look inside the patient. This scan showed where a needle needed to go. The PUMA 200 robot slid the needle into the patient's brain. It took a tissue sample. The **biopsy** was tested for cancer.

A robot called PROBOT was first used in 1988. Before the surgery, scans were made. They were of the patient's prostate gland. This gland is below a man's bladder. The doctor studied the scans. The robot would make cuts inside the gland. The doctor noted where to make the cuts. He programmed the robot. The robot reached the gland. The doctor watched PROBOT work. He could take over if needed. The robot made cut after cut. Each cut was exact. This was the perfect task for a robot.

Around the same time, ROBODOC was developed to help with hip surgeries. Hip

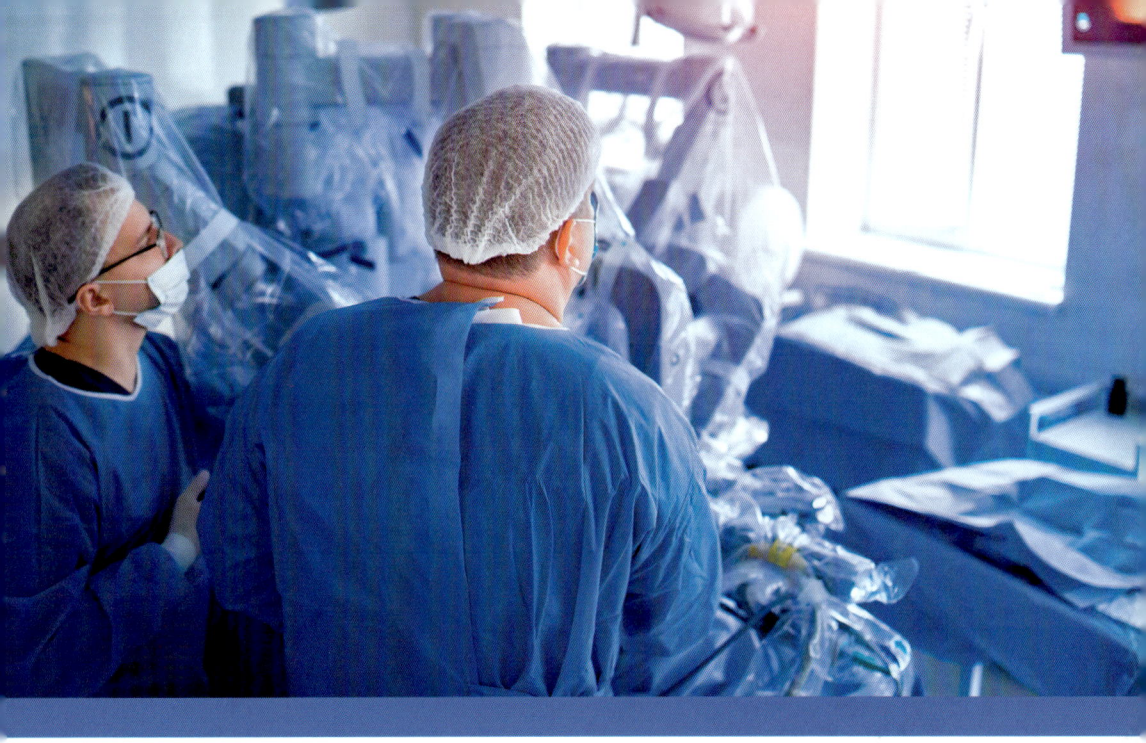

Over the last few decades, robots have become more common in operating rooms.

replacement is difficult. The surgeon cuts holes in the **femur**. This is the person's upper leg bone. The holes hold part of the new hip. Handmade cuts vary in size. Some are uneven. Dr. William Bargar worked at the University of California, Davis. He built ROBODOC. In 1992, the robot was first used on a human. It made perfect cuts in the femur.

LAPAROSCOPIC SURGERY

Laparoscopes are used in robotic surgery. A laparoscope is a thin tool. It is like a telescope with a light. It is very flexible. Doctors slip it into the patient. This is done through a small cut. These small cuts heal faster than larger incisions. Doctors can use laparoscopes to look inside a person's abdomen. A doctor can work on a person's beating heart. Doctors use them with robots.

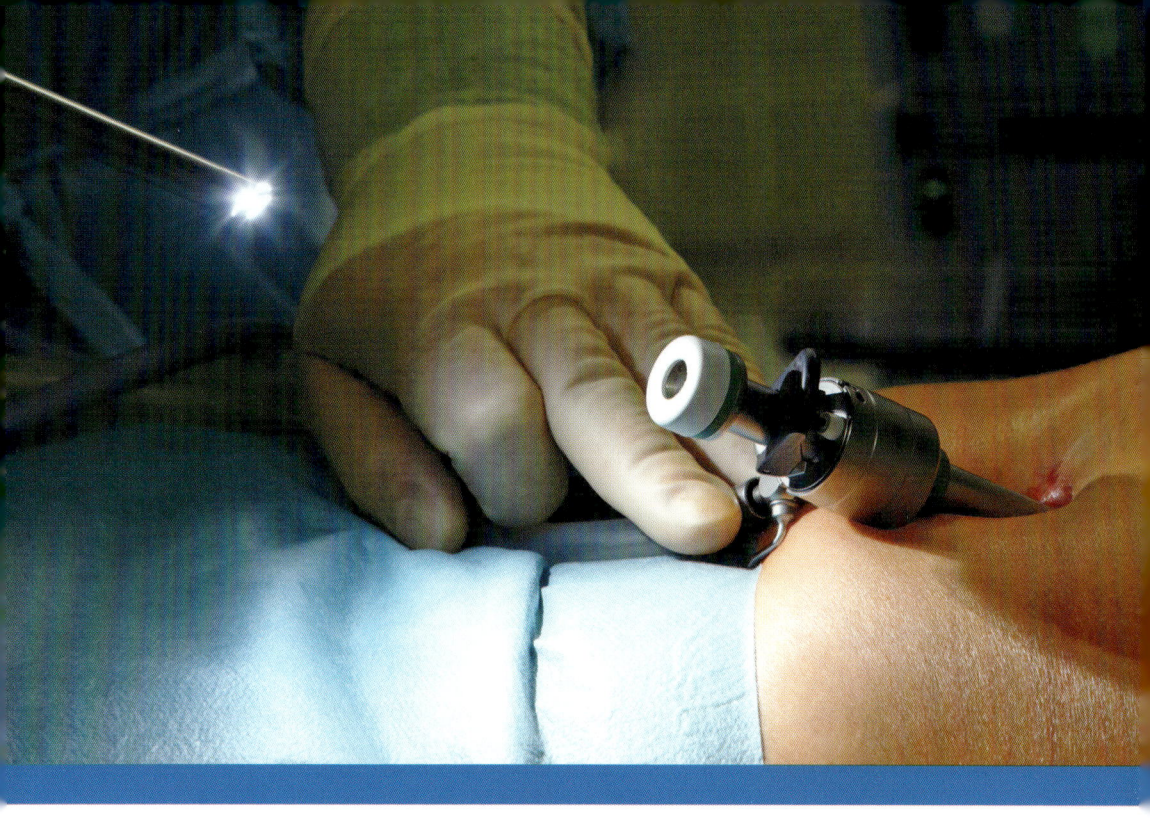

Laparoscopes are useful tools for safer surgeries.

In the late 1990s, several robotic systems were built. They were made for laparoscopic surgery. One was the da Vinci system. Today, it is the most widely used surgical robot. It has three or four arms. These arms have wrist-like joints. They can

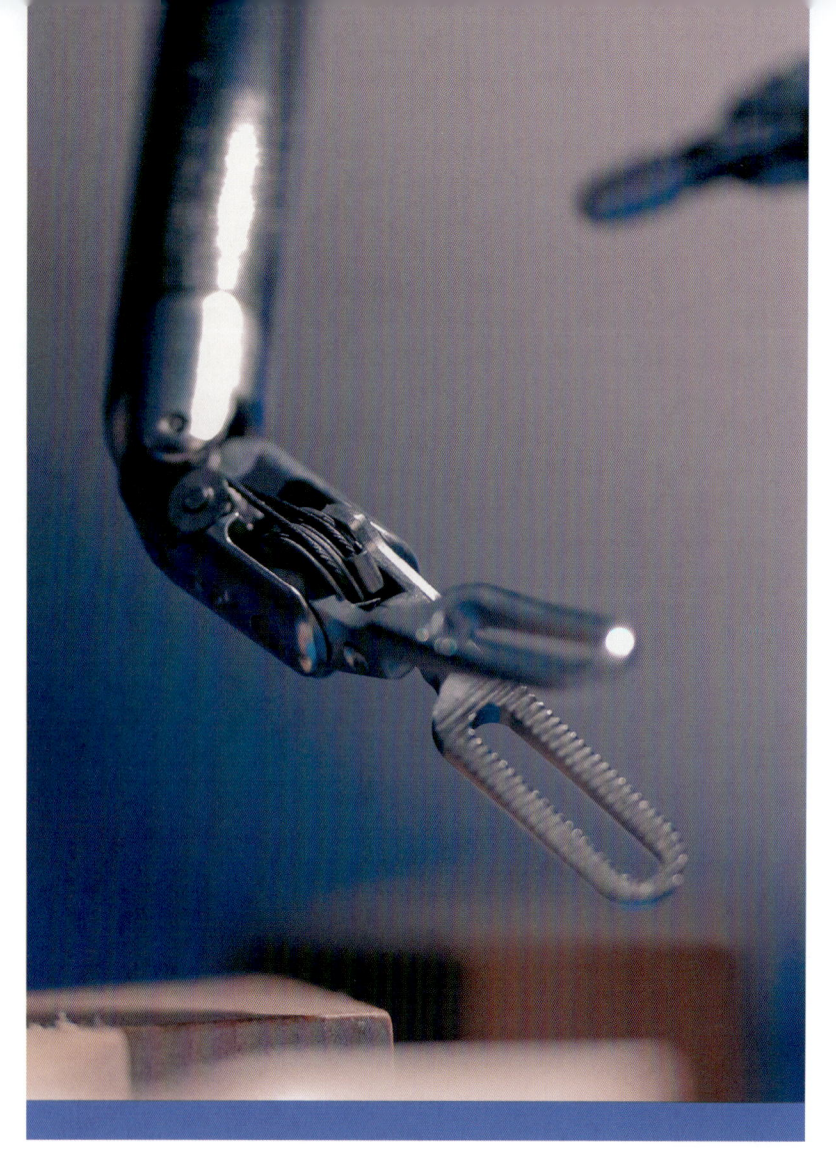

The ends of a surgery robot's arms may hold small, delicate instruments.

reach where a doctor cannot. "The surgeon's role is totally different now," says Dr. Andrew Wagner.[2] He is a director at

GROWTH OF ROBOTIC SURGERY

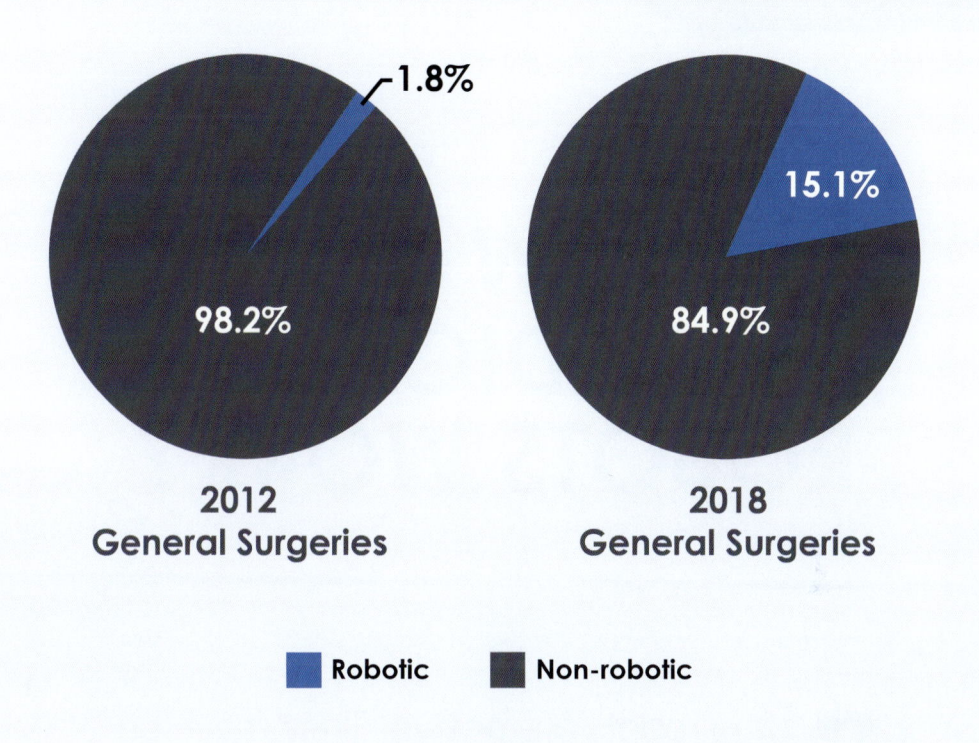

2012 General Surgeries: 1.8% Robotic, 98.2% Non-robotic

2018 General Surgeries: 15.1% Robotic, 84.9% Non-robotic

Source: Kyle H. Sheetz, MD, MSc; Jake Claflin, BS; Justin B. Dimick, MD, MPH, "Trends in the Adoption of Robotic Surgery for Common Surgical Procedures," JAMA Network Open, January 10, 2020. https://jamanetwork.com.

The use of robots in surgery became much more widespread in the 2010s.

Beth Israel Deaconess Medical Center. This is in Boston, Massachusetts. Robots are changing today's hospitals.

CHAPTER TWO

HOW DO MEDICAL ROBOTS WORK?

Some robots are **active**. They move on their own. One example is a delivery robot. It is given a task. It might take blood samples to a lab. It could take meals to patients. Its computer program tells it where to go.

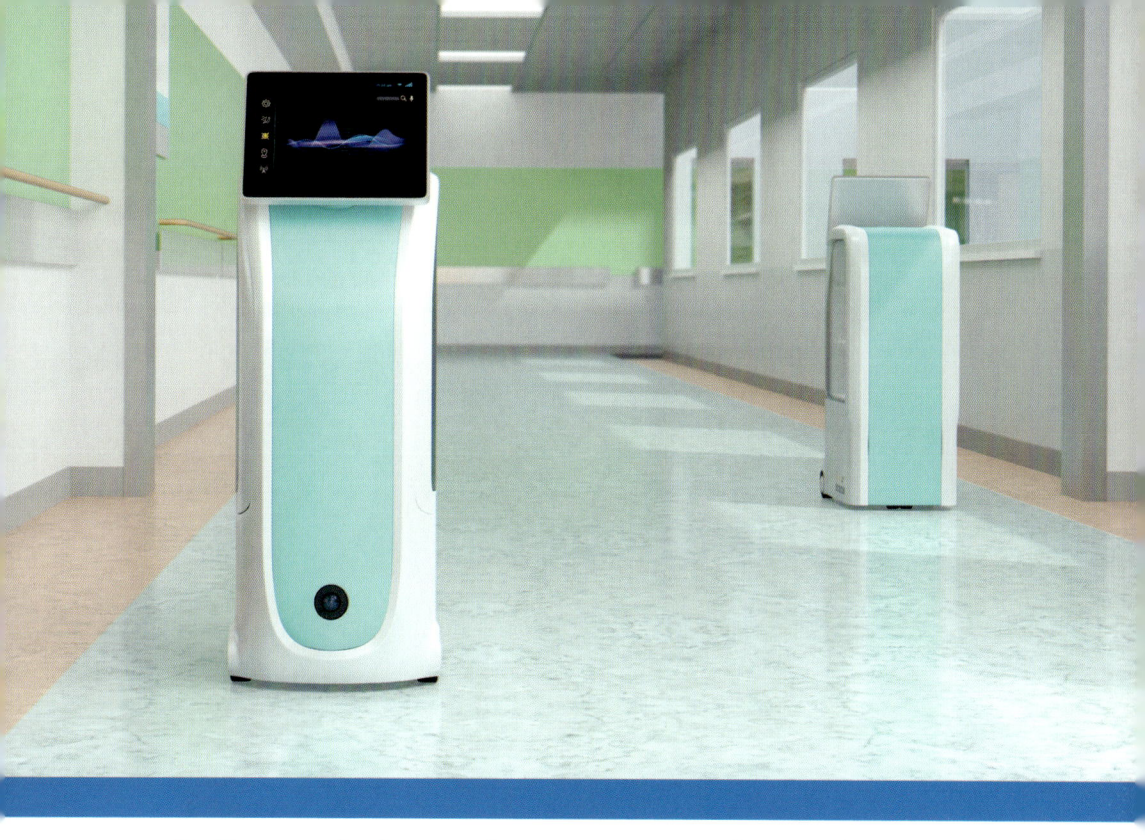

Delivery robots may be programmed to navigate independently around a hospital.

Other robots are **passive**. A person directs each move this robot makes. Surgery robots often work this way. When a surgery robot cuts out a tumor, it does not move on its own. The doctor uses

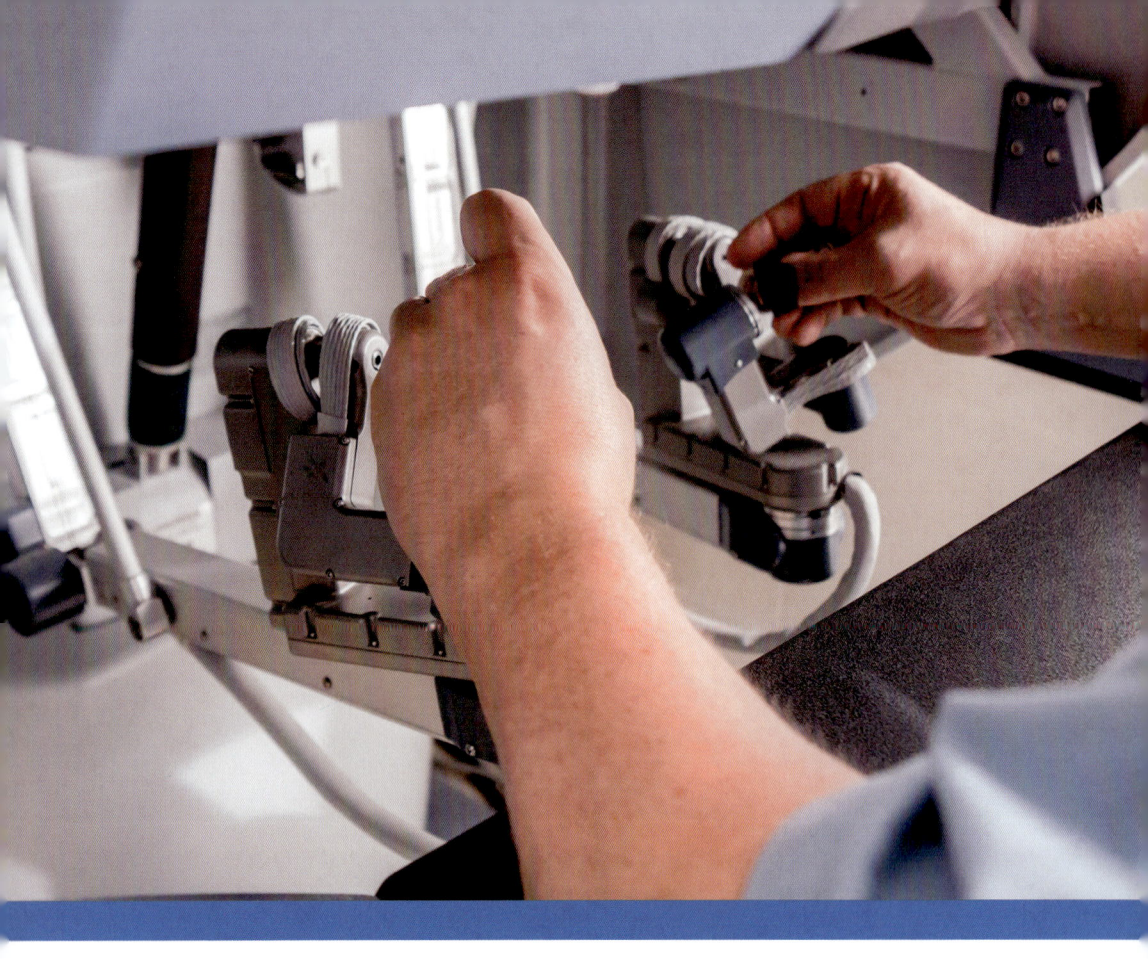

Surgeons control passive robots using hand controllers.

controllers to move the robot. Some robots are both active and passive. It depends on the job the robot is doing at that time. In one surgery, a robot may begin by being active. The robot moves through the person's mouth. It moves down the person's throat. Or it might move up the intestine. Then it stops. The doctor takes over. The robot becomes passive.

SENSORS

All robots need sensors. Sensors give them information about the world around them. They need this information to do their jobs. There are many types of sensors.

Some robots have cameras. A camera lets a robot see. The doctor can see this view on a screen. She can see a tumor or a person's heart. The camera gives the doctor an up-close view.

A robot's camera may be able to measure heat. One robot with a heat-sensitive camera is named MITRA. MITRA works at Fortis Hospital. This hospital is in Bangalore, India. MITRA uses its camera to take people's temperatures. In 2020, MITRA helped screen patients for symptoms of the disease COVID-19. This helped people get the help they needed.

MITRA uses other sensors to do its job as well. MITRA needs to speak with people. Microphones let it hear spoken words. A computer processes the words and

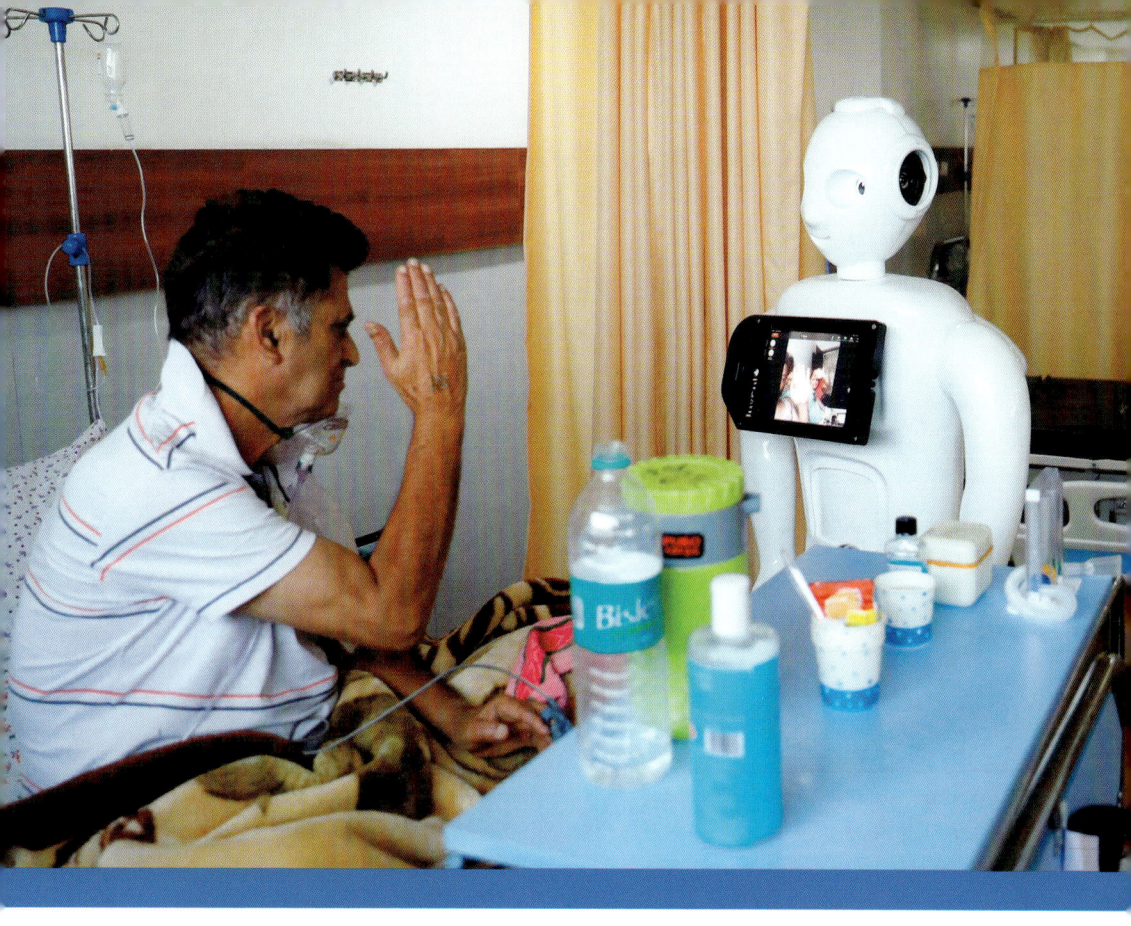

A MITRA robot helps a patient near New Delhi, India.

plans a response. Speakers allow MITRA to respond.

TUG is a delivery robot. It moves through busy hallways. It needs to know what is in the halls. It uses heat sensors. Heat sensors see body heat. This keeps TUG from running into people. TUG also uses laser sensors. Laser light bounces off objects and back to TUG. These reflections tell the robot something is in its way. It can steer

MAKING MITRA

Invento Robotics built MITRA in 2017. It had to overcome many problems. One problem was the robot's footprint. This is the area the robot stands on. If the footprint is too small, the robot might tip over. It could fall and hurt someone. But the footprint cannot take up too much room. The team had to find the right size. They also had to teach the robot to move. An uneven floor means it must move slowly to avoid falling over. Being stable is a big challenge for moving robots.

around objects. Staff members use touch pads to scroll through menus and tell TUG what to do.

ROBOT MUSCLES

People use muscles to move. A muscle can get longer. This happens when a person stretches. A muscle can get shorter. This happens when a person tenses the muscle. Both actions are needed to walk or sit. Both are needed to lift objects.

Robots need to move. But they do not have muscles. They use motors instead. Some robots have servo motors. These motors are good for quick movements.

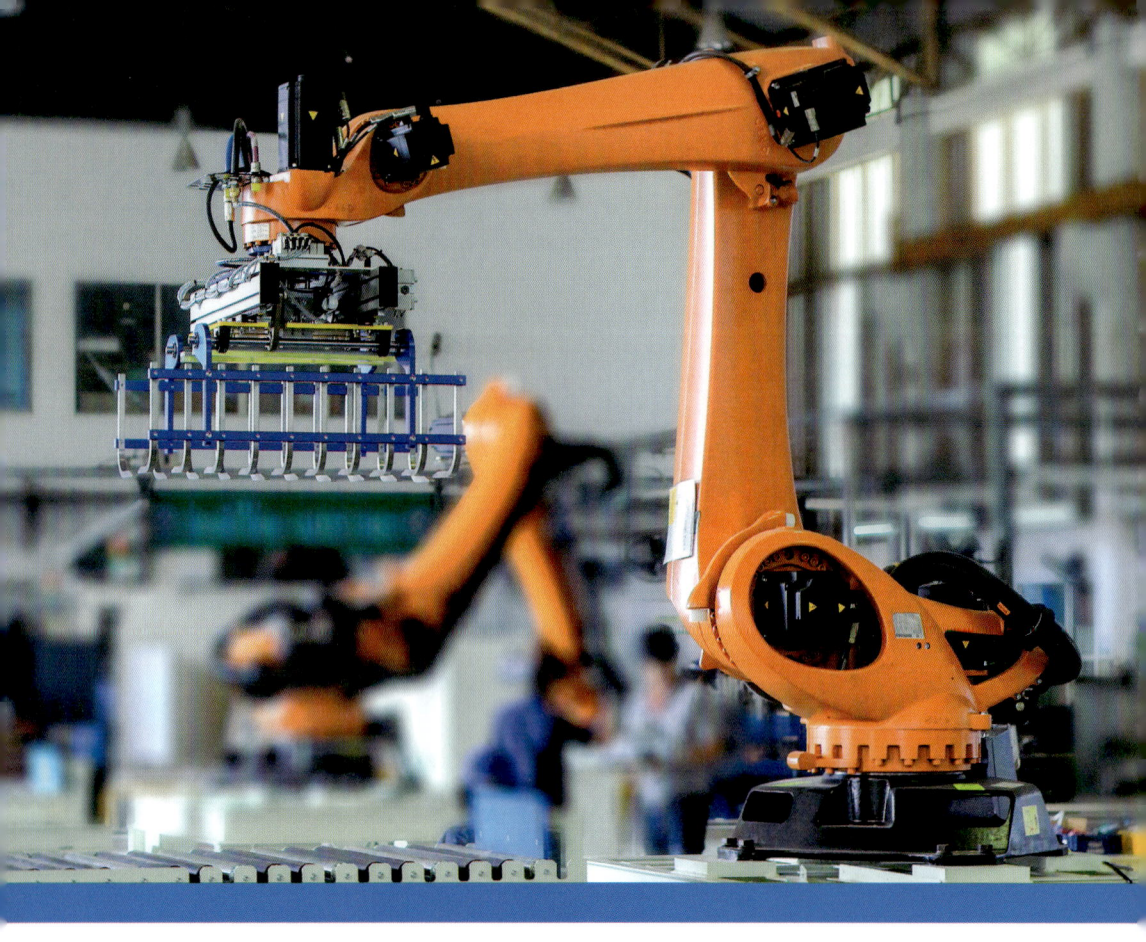

The motors in robotic arms can be capable of amazing strength.

They are strong. They can do the same thing again and again. Servo motors are used for robotic arms. They are used for surgical robots and in labs.

Robots also use stepper motors. These motors also work quickly. But they can move in shorter steps. They do not move as far as fast. They are better for smaller movements.

Many factors go into picking the right motor. A motor for surgery must be small. It must be able to make precise movements. A motor used in a lab must be quiet. A motor for a delivery robot needs to respond quickly if the robot has to stop. Hospitals are busy places. Someone may step in front of the robot.

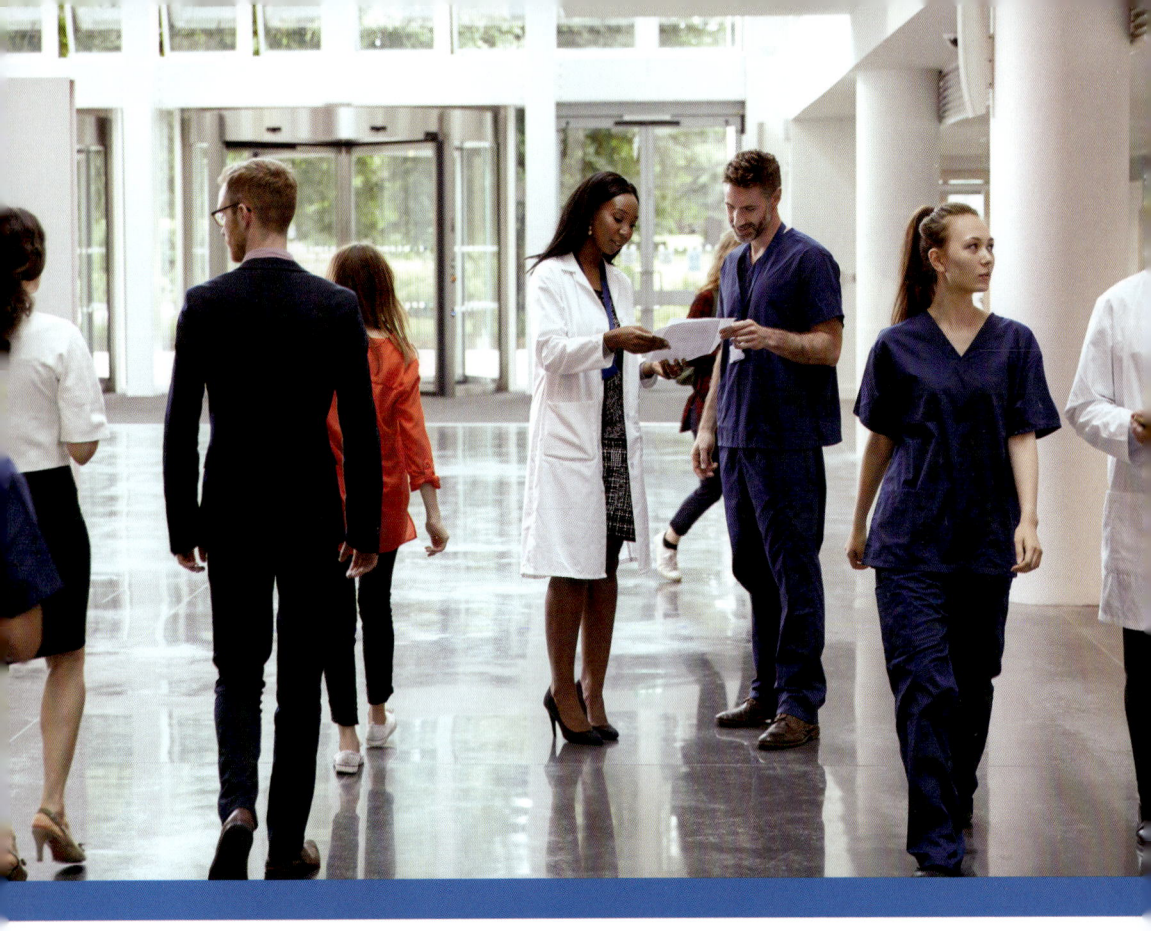

A busy hospital can be a challenging place for a robot to operate.

ROBOT BRAINS

All robots use computer programs to function. The programs tell them what to do. This is how the robots carry out their jobs. A hospital worker loads a TUG.

The worker starts the program. The program runs. The TUG goes to the right place. It works automatically.

In surgery, a doctor uses controllers. But there is still a program running. The program turns the motions of the controllers into the robot's movements. The program makes the movements smooth and small. There is none of the shaking that human hands might have. "It completely reduces the tremor," said Dr. Bahareh Nejad.[3] She is in charge of robotic surgery. She works at University of California, Davis Medical Center.

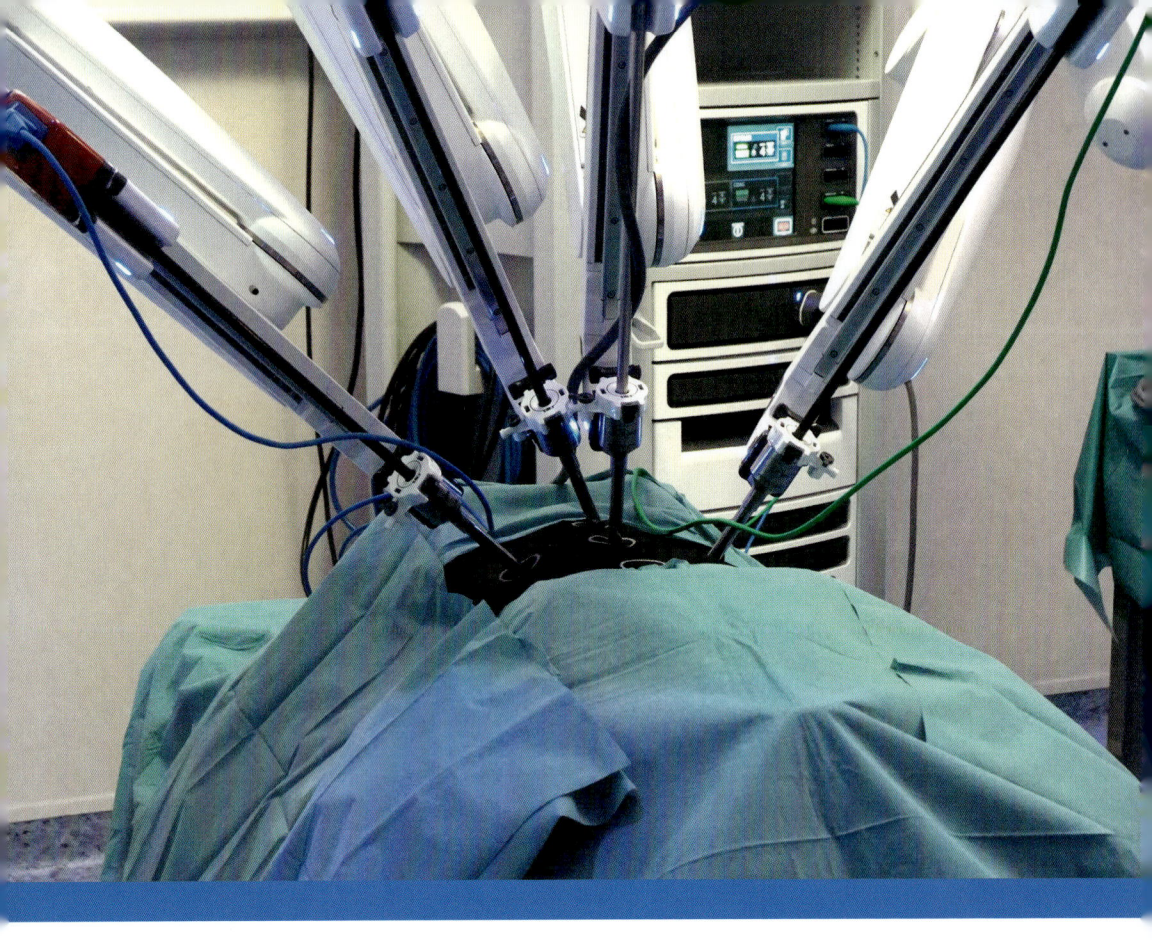

Surgery robots can make tiny, precise movements.

Active robots have complex programs. MITRA has to talk with people. It asks what they need. It gives them directions. "You will have people speaking different languages," said Amit Tripathy.[4] He is a project manager at Invento Robotics. This company builds MITRA. MITRA was programmed to speak several languages. It has to tell different languages apart. It has to know which language to speak. Its program is very complex.

KEEPING CLEAN

Robots in hospitals come into contact with people. These robots must be sterile. This means they must be free of germs. Surgical robots wear special sleeves. The sleeves can be washed. The tools used by the robot must also be cleaned. Surgical tools are washed in a special machine. It is called an autoclave.

CHAPTER THREE

HOW ARE DOCTORS USING ROBOTS TODAY?

Hospital robots do many jobs. This includes surgery. Surgical robots help remove organs. The robot can help take out a gallbladder. It might remove an appendix. A person can live without these organs. But an infection in one of them can

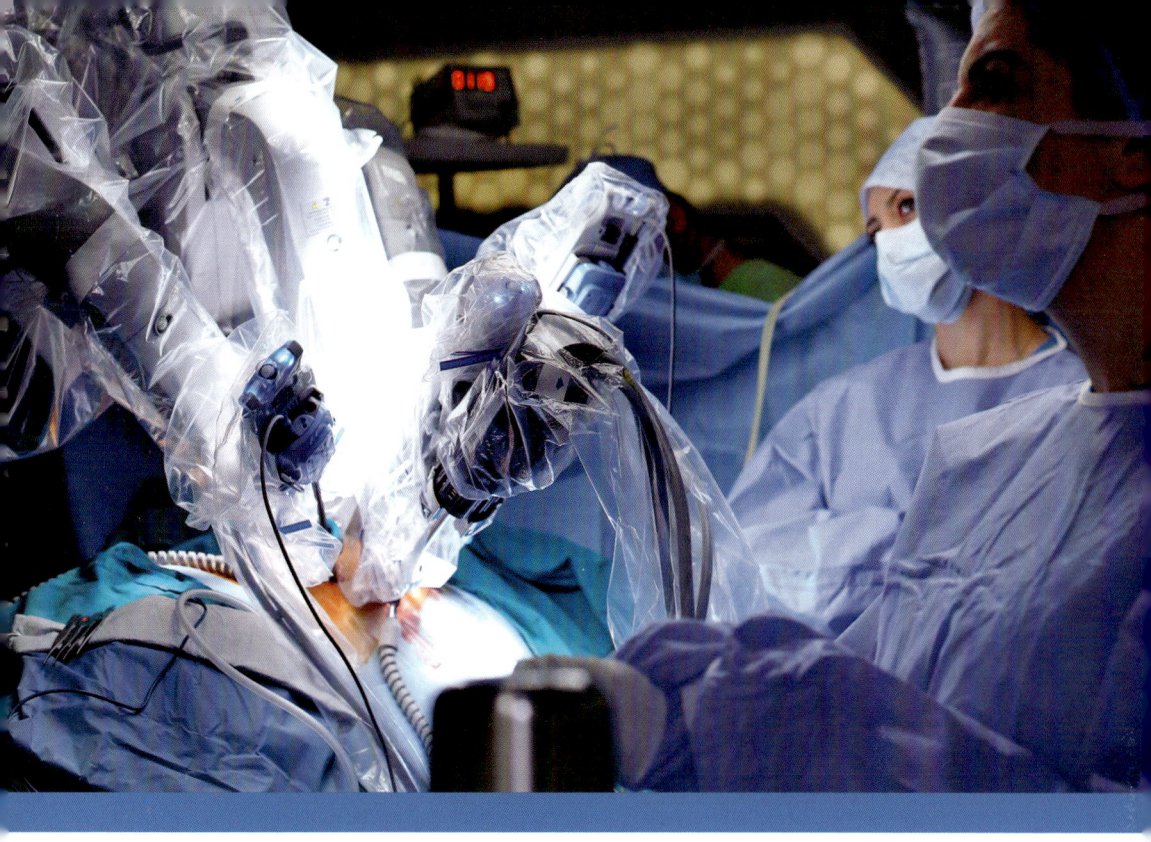

Surgical robots are often covered in plastic to prevent the spread of germs.

cause serious problems. The infected organ must be removed.

Surgical robots also take biopsies. A biopsy is a tiny sample. It will be tested for disease. The disease might be a cancer.

It could be an infection. A robot can take a sample from the brain. It can also sample the colon. This is part of the digestive system. If cancer is found, sometimes a robot helps cut it out.

Robots also help make repairs. They can help fix a heart valve. A robot can even help replace a valve. Robots help in eye surgery.

HIGH COSTS

Robotic surgery has many advantages. But there is one big drawback. It costs more than non-robotic surgery. First, the hospital must buy the robotic system. In 2020, the da Vinci system cost $2 million. Each doctor must then be trained to use the robots. This also costs money. These costs make the surgeries more expensive for patients.

This includes cataract surgery. The robot makes a tiny cut in the person's eye. The lens is taken out of the eye. The doctor replaces it with a new lens. Small cuts mean that patients heal quickly.

RADIATION

Some robots help treat cancer. One of them is the CyberKnife. It is a robotic system. It is not a knife. It does not cut into the patient. Instead it zaps the tumor. It uses a beam of radiation.

The radiation source is on a robotic arm. The doctor moves the arm into place. The CyberKnife sends out a thin beam. This thin

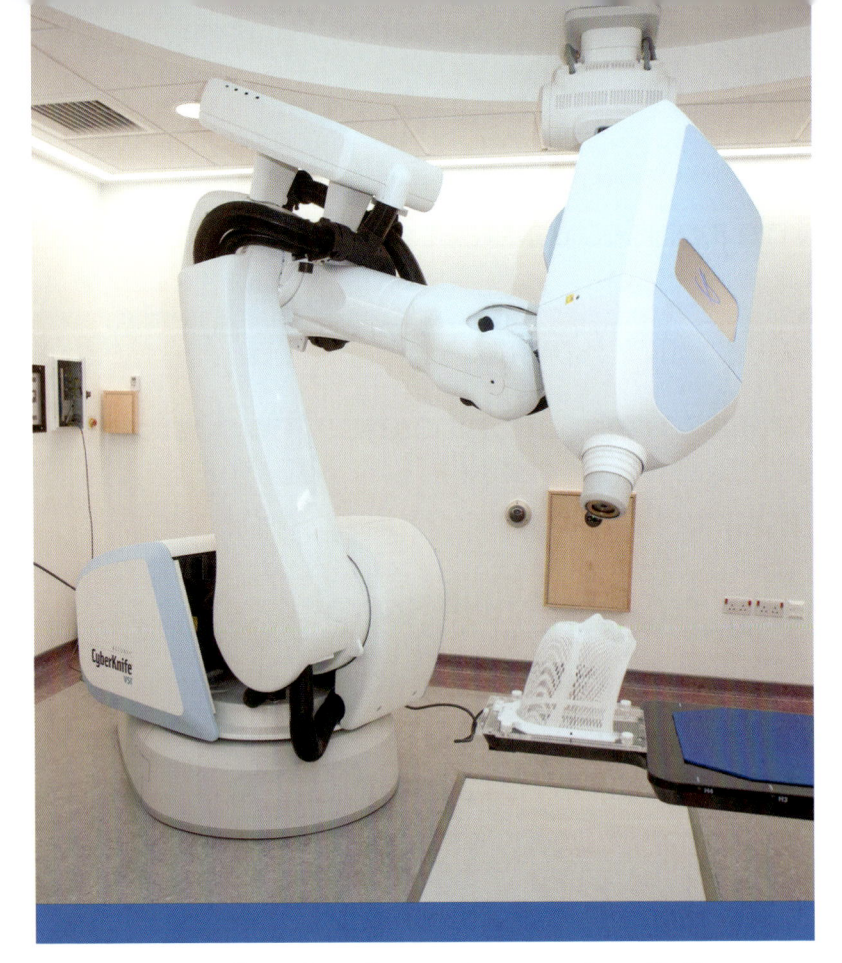

The CyberKnife robot fires a beam of radiation at just the right point inside a patient.

beam is aimed at an exact location. Then the arm shifts. The robot sends out more radiation. Again and again, the arm shifts. There is another zap of radiation. The robot can often reach every side of a tumor.

Patients move during treatment. They breathe. They shift. They relax. This moves the tumor, too. The robot tracks the tumor. It adjusts its aim. The radiation stays focused on the tumor. This is important. Radiation can harm healthy organs. But healthy organs and skin get very little radiation with CyberKnife. This makes treatment easier on the patient. The patient has fewer side effects.

DELIVERY

Hospitals are often very big. Some have several buildings. Hallways stretch from end to end. It is a long walk to deliver supplies.

This may not seem important. But patients need three meals a day. Medicines are delivered throughout the hospital. Blood and other samples must go to the lab. Laundry must be brought from place to place. This all adds up. Delivery robots free people up to do other jobs.

A delivery robot can carry hundreds of medicines at once. It can call an elevator. It takes the elevator to the correct floor. Then it reaches the nurse's station. It calls for a nurse. The nurse puts his finger on the sensor. If the robot recognizes the nurse's fingerprint, the correct bin opens. The nurse

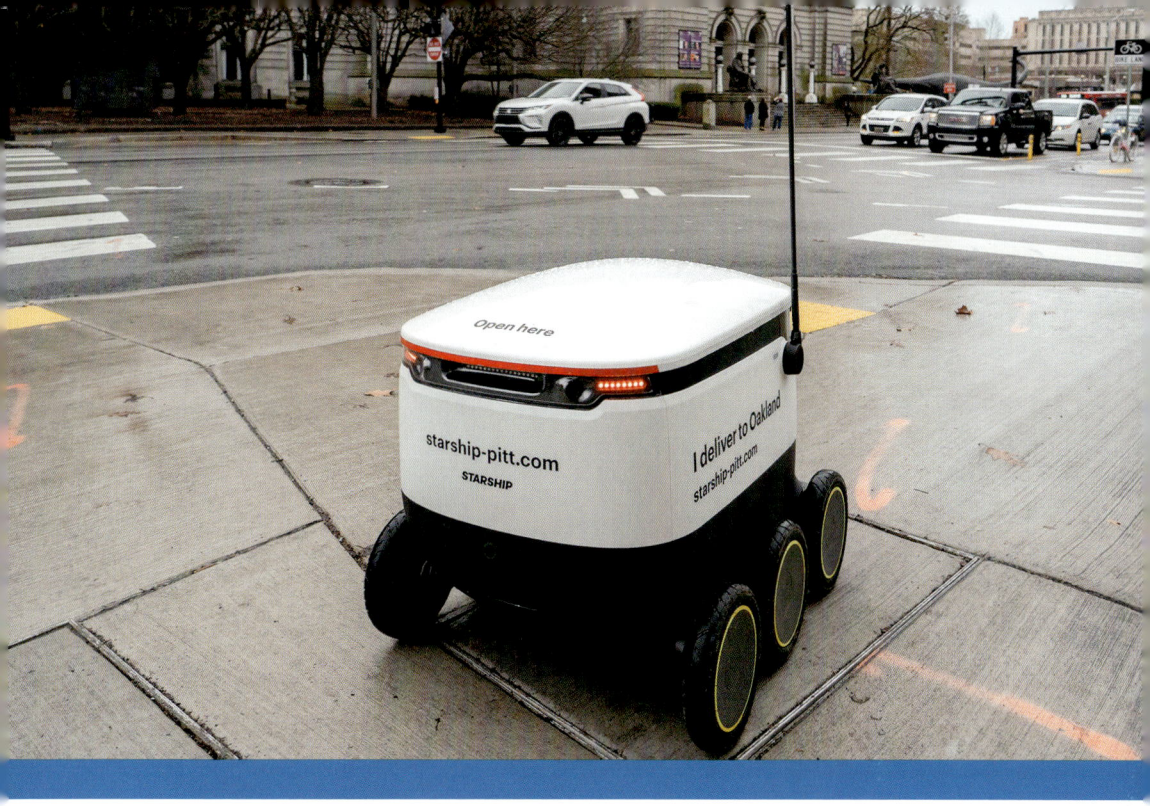

Delivery robots are now used in many places, including hospitals, warehouses, and even city streets.

takes out the medicine. Using robots to deliver medicines cuts down on errors.

The staff can check the robot's progress. It is similar to how people can track mail or packages. "This is just bringing it into the hospital," said Mary Jane Turner.[5] Turner is a

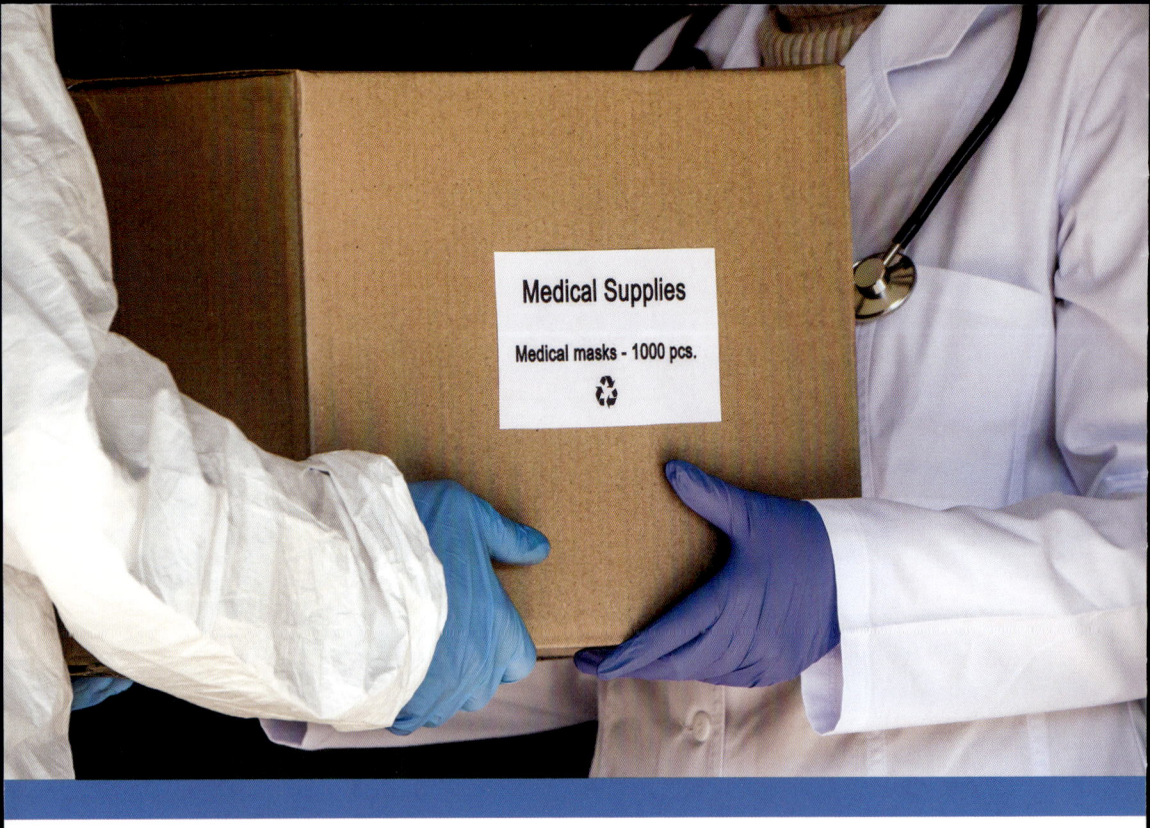

Using robots for deliveries can free up valuable staff time.

pharmacy specialist. She works at MedStar Washington. This hospital is in Washington, DC. "People know when their packages are going to arrive at home, so why shouldn't we know where our medications are at all times?" she asks.[6]

CLEANING ROBOTS

It is hard to keep hospitals clean. Sick people bring in germs. Some germs are hard to kill. An estimated one in thirty-one patients gets an infection while in the hospital. Researchers have found a new way to kill germs. People cannot see ultraviolet (UV) light. But it kills many germs.

Henry Ford Hospital is in Detroit, Michigan. This hospital uses two robots to clean, or disinfect, patient rooms. The staff calls the robots Zappy and Germinator. Jennifer Ritz is a nurse at this hospital. She talked to a writer about using the robots.

"Once it's placed in the room and started, the head pops up and turns around while the UV rays are pulsating throughout the room," says Ritz.[7] After one round, someone enters the room. This person flips the mattress on the bed. The program is run again. The robot bathes the room in UV light. The light kills germs. The room is clean. The robots remember which rooms they cleaned. They know how long it took to clean each room.

These robots have not replaced other types of cleaning. They added another layer. Hospitals still hire other staff to do other

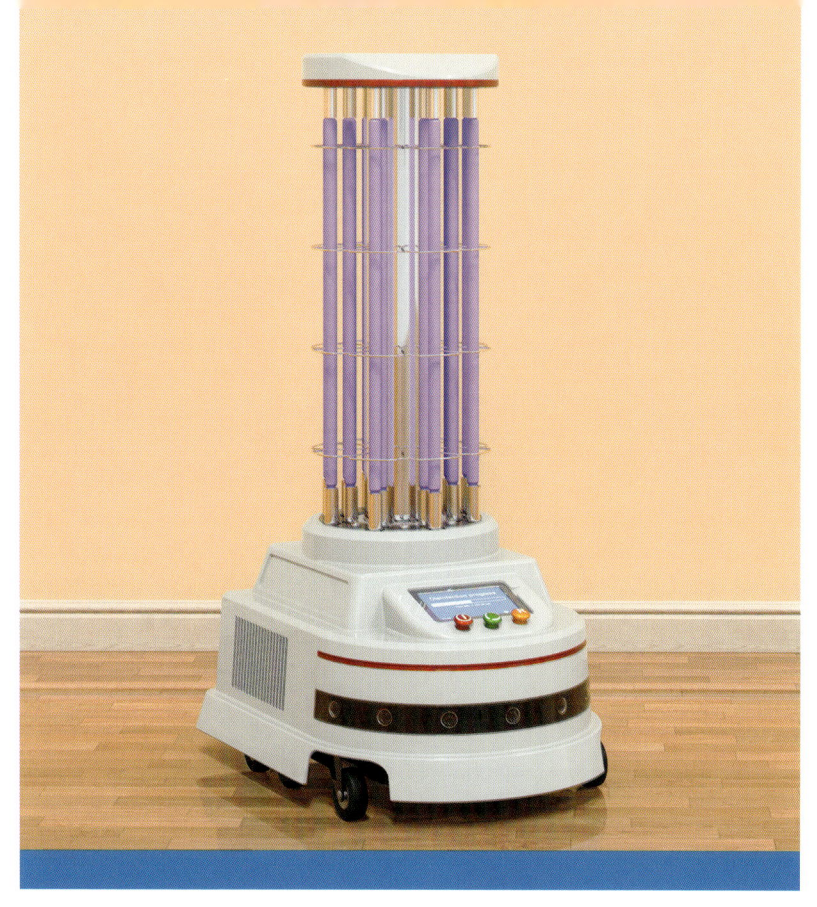

Cleaning robots in hospitals offer an extra layer of protection against infection.

kinds of cleaning. And they also hire people to work with the robots.

REHAB ROBOTS

Robots also work in **rehabilitation**, or rehab. In rehab, a patient does a set of exercises. The exercises help the patient get strong. They help the patient heal. A person with a broken arm does one set of exercises. A person who had a heart attack does another. Each exercise targets a problem.

Dotty Attie had a stroke. A stroke happens when blood flow to the brain is

JENNIE

Sometimes a sick person must give up their pets. Jennie can cheer them up. Jennie is a robot puppy. It is made by Tombot. It lies on a cushion. It turns its head, lifts its ears, and wags its tail. Jennie looks friendly. But it does not need food or water. No one has to take it for a walk. Yet it gives support and comfort.

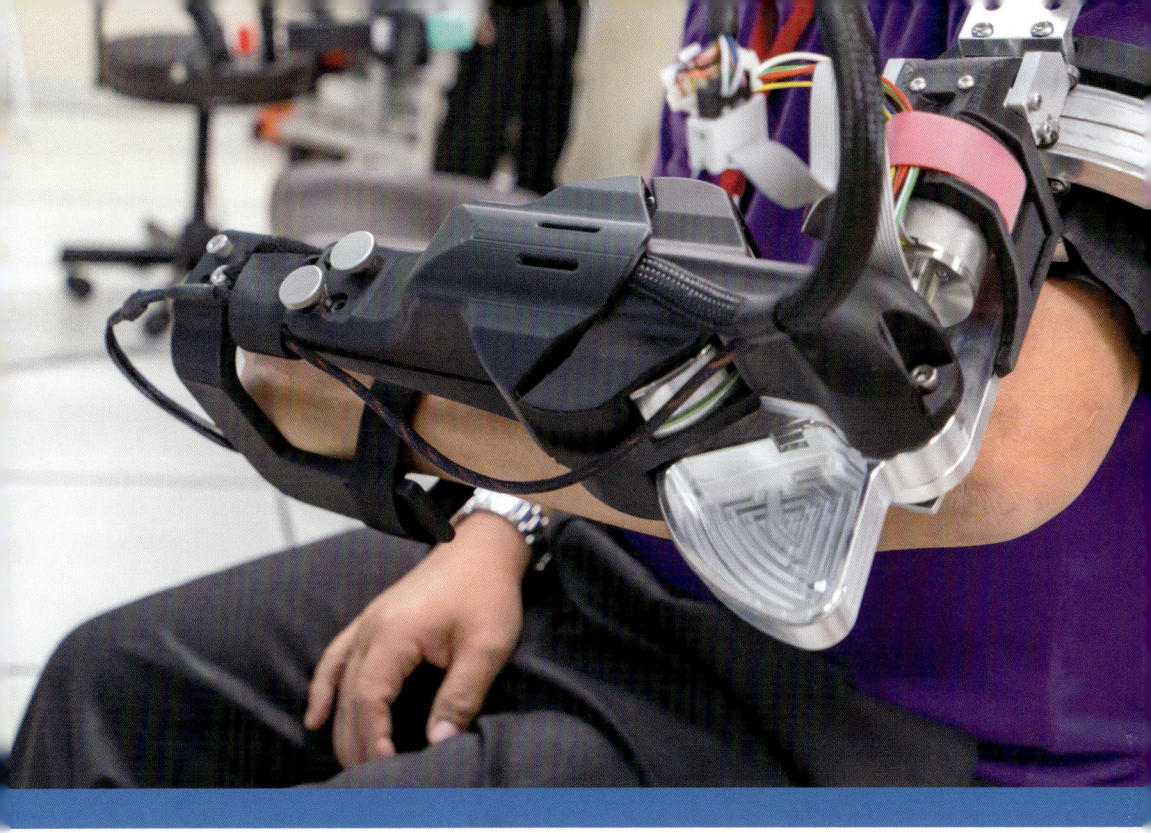

Robotic arms can help people who are rehabilitating after injury or illness.

interrupted. It causes brain damage. Attie lost some movement in her hand. She went to rehab. Her hand was fitted into a robot. She opened her hand as far as she could. Then the robot took over. It opened her hand the rest of the way. She and the robot

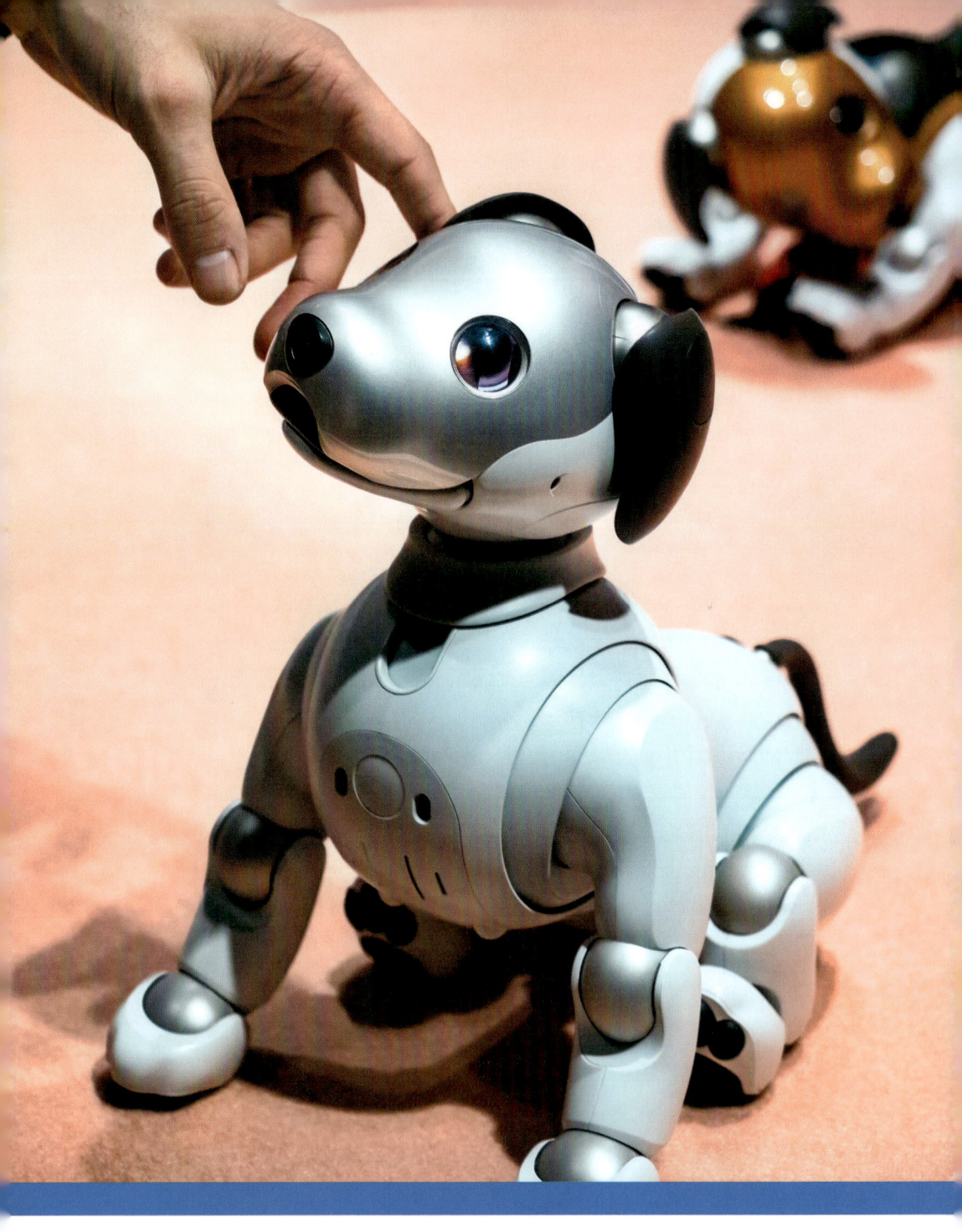

Robotic pets can be welcome companions for patients in hospitals.

did this again and again. The repetition retrained her brain.

Robotic pets also offer therapy. One robot is called Paro. Paro looks like a baby seal. Paro bats its eyes and coos. It turns its head when the patient speaks to it. It looks like it is alive. Young patients find the robot comforting. They become less worried. This makes it easier for them to heal.

CHAPTER FOUR

WHAT'S NEXT FOR ROBOTICS IN HEALTH CARE?

Robots have jobs to do. In the future, they will do even more. Many jobs will be in hospitals. Robots will see more patients. Many of these robots will be tele-robots. These robots helped during the COVID-19 pandemic in 2020. Tele-robots

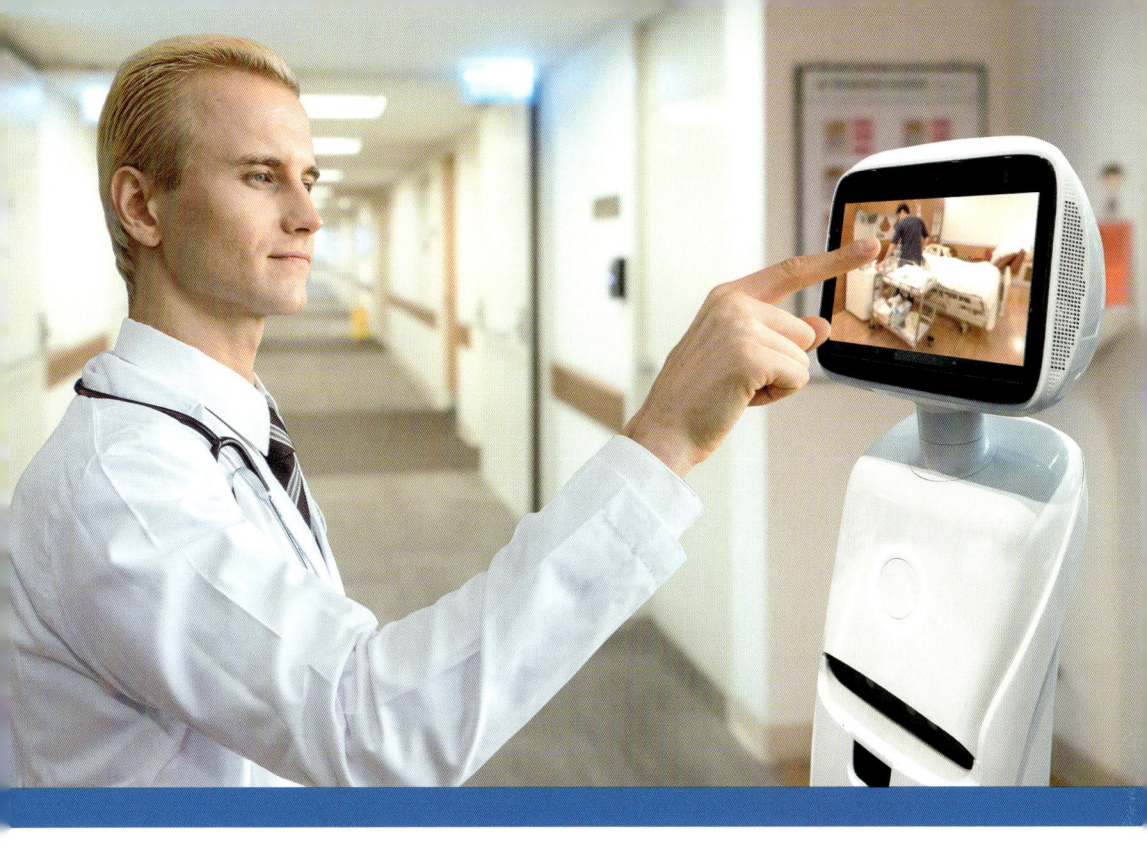

As technology advances, robots are likely to take on more roles in hospitals.

help people talk to each other. They are like video calls. The robot has a screen and a camera. The patient can see the nurse. The nurse can see the patient. They can talk.

These robots do many other things as well. They take the patient's temperature.

They can help nurses check the patient in other ways. Some patients are infectious. This means that they can make other people sick. A nurse could be at risk. But the nurse is in another room. The nurse controls the robot and stays safe. These robots will reduce the spread of disease.

SMALL-TOWN MEDICINE

Small-town hospitals often employ fewer doctors. They may not have a cancer doctor. They may not have a doctor who knows about eyes. But a tele-robot could help. A doctor might be in a distant city. She could consult at several small-town hospitals. This could give people in the towns better health care without having to travel far from home.

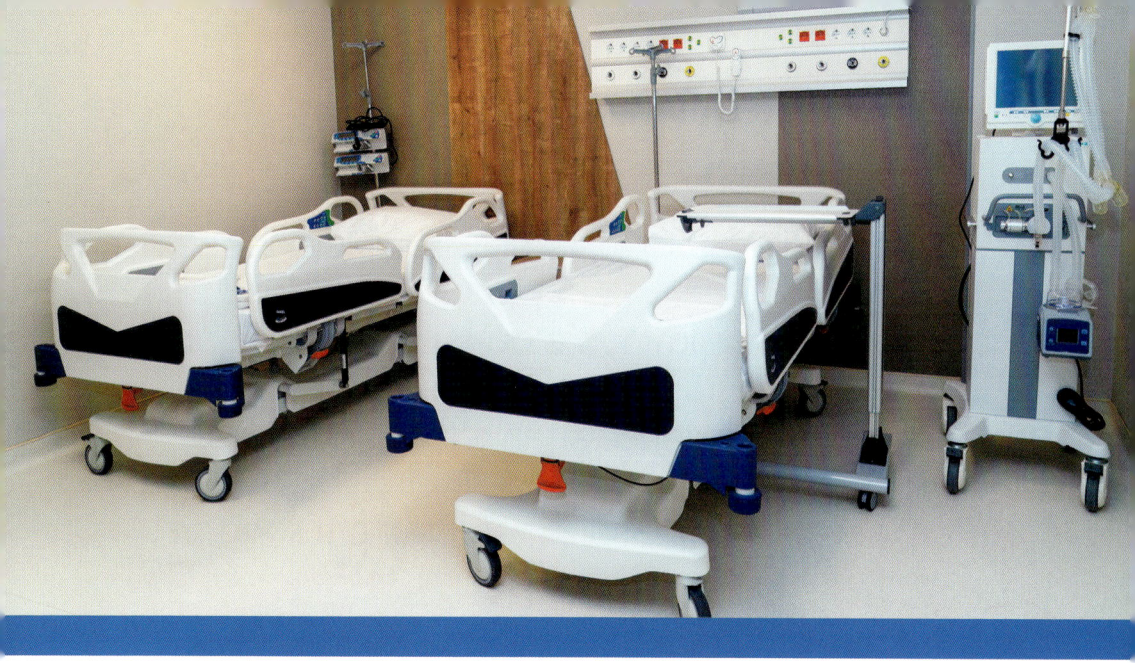

Robots will need to be small and nimble to navigate cramped hospital rooms.

MITRA helped during the COVID-19 pandemic. But not all robots are ready for wide use. When some robots do not work right, the problem can be hard to find. Hospital staff need to be trained. They need to learn how to find and fix problems.

The robots also need to be smaller. Many robots in use today have large bases. This makes them stable. A stable robot is less likely to tip over. But there are many places they cannot fit. This can be a problem if hospital rooms are full of equipment.

MORE ROBOTIC SURGERY

In April 2019, Dr. Pierre Dupont reported a victory. He is head of pediatric cardiac bioengineering at Boston Children's Hospital. This hospital is in Boston, Massachusetts. Dupont works on children's hearts.

A leaky heart valve is life-threatening. When a valve leaks, the heart does not

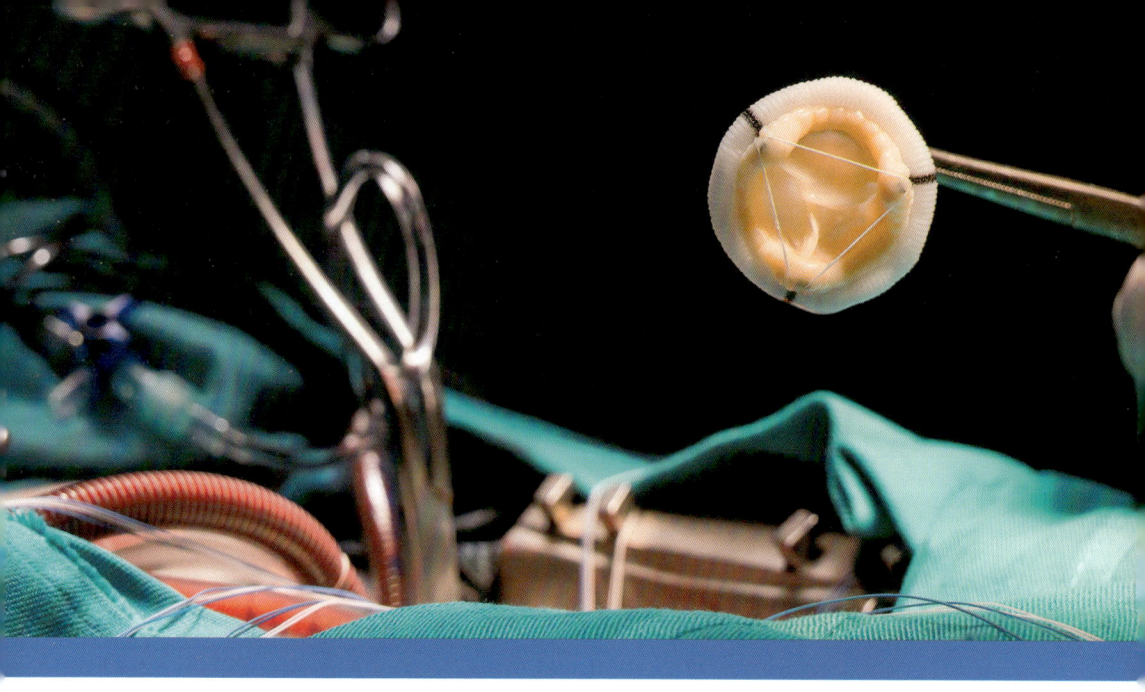

Heart valve surgery can be tricky. Robotic catheters offer a way to make it simpler.

work right. The person's muscles and organs do not get enough blood. A leaky valve can be replaced. The new valve is often artificial. Sometimes leaks form around these valves. The leaks must be plugged. This requires surgery. The surgery involves opening the patient's chest. Bones must be cut. It takes a long time to heal.

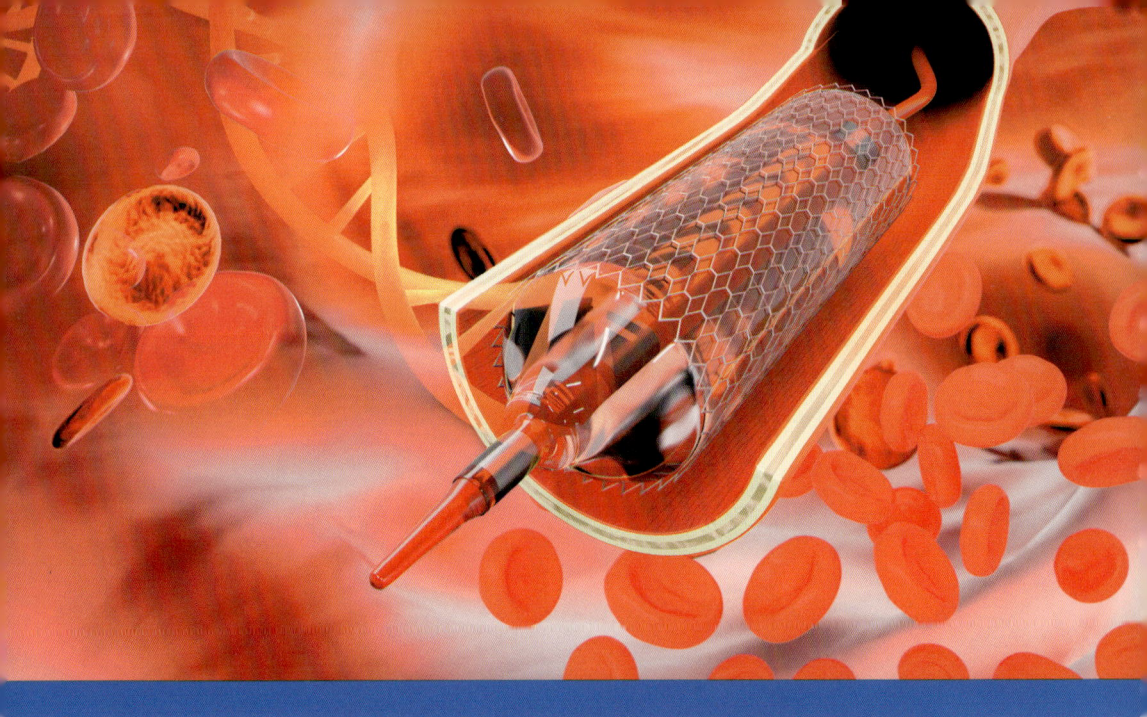

Catheters are often used to evaluate and treat the heart.

Dupont worked with a team of doctors. They used a robotic catheter. A catheter is a tube. The robotic catheter was active. It moved by itself. It followed the heart wall. To do this, it had a sensor. The sensor works like a cat's whiskers. It can feel the heart wall. This kept the robot moving in the right direction. The sensor can also feel the valve. The robot stopped at the valve. Then the doctor took over. Doctors pushed a plug through the tube. It sealed the leak.

    This robot is not fast. It takes just as long as a human doctor. But the robot can see in the heart. A doctor cannot. A doctor needs scans to see in the heart. Scans require weak radiation, which can do damage. The robot needs no scans. The child's heart is not exposed to radiation. There is another problem with scanners. Not all hospitals have them. Any doctor can use the robot, meaning more children could be helped.

MICROSCOPIC MEDICINE

Scientists are also working on very small robots that can operate inside the body. These robots can move themselves. They can be used to treat diseases.

One type of robot is known as a micromotor. Scientists at the University of California, Berkeley, have tested these. They fed the micromotors to mice. The micromotors were tubes coated with the mineral zinc. The mice swallowed the micromotors, which reached their stomachs. Zinc reacts with stomach acid. When this happened, bubbles formed.

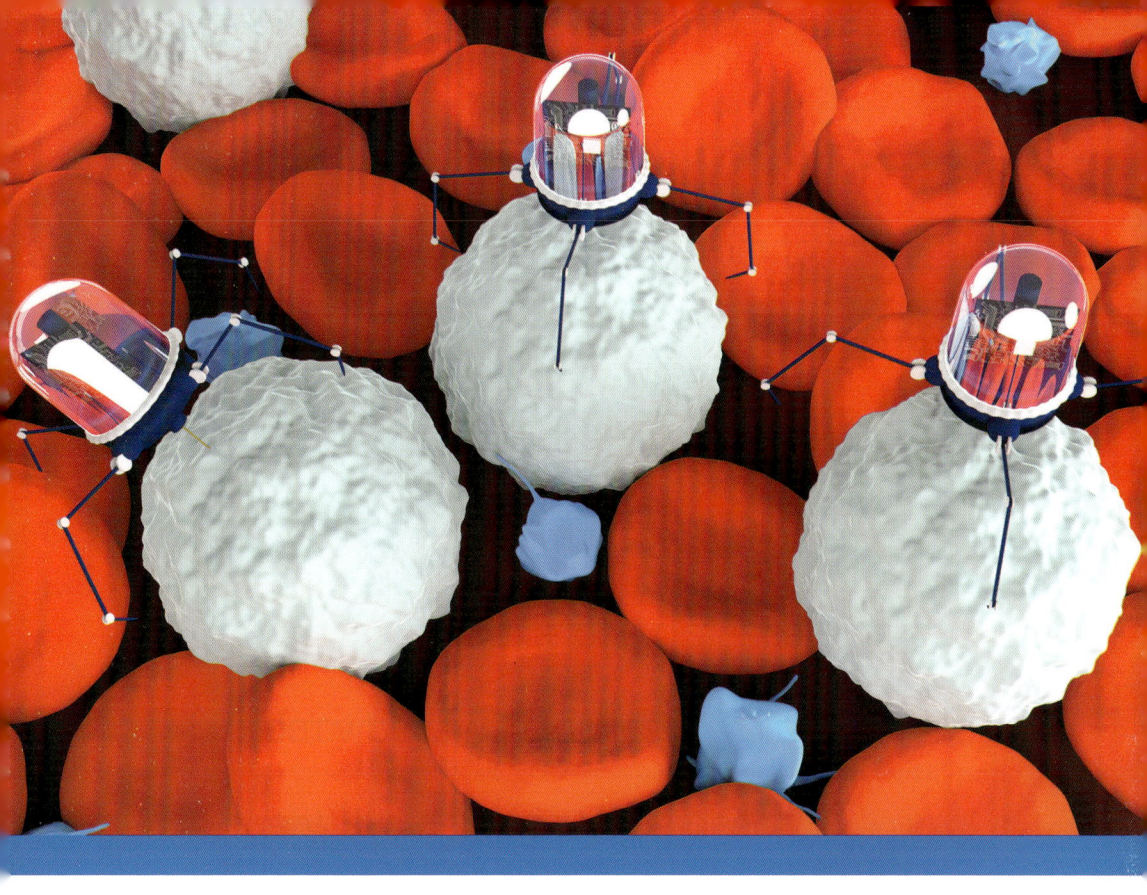

Tiny robots used in the body are mostly science fiction today, but researchers are working to turn them into reality.

The bubbles were forced out of the tubes. The tubes worked like jets. They moved through the stomach acid. They got to the stomach wall and lodged in its mucus coating. The micromotors left material on the stomach wall. In the future, tubes like these could carry medicines into the stomach.

Micromotors face a few problems. One problem is fuel. Most micromotors carry fuel. These micromotors contain the metal platinum. The fuel is most often hydrogen peroxide. It reacts with the platinum and forms bubbles. But hydrogen peroxide makes people sick when swallowed. A new fuel will be needed. Or the micromotors can be made from something else. Micromotors can be made with zinc, as with the mouse experiment. Zinc reacts with stomach

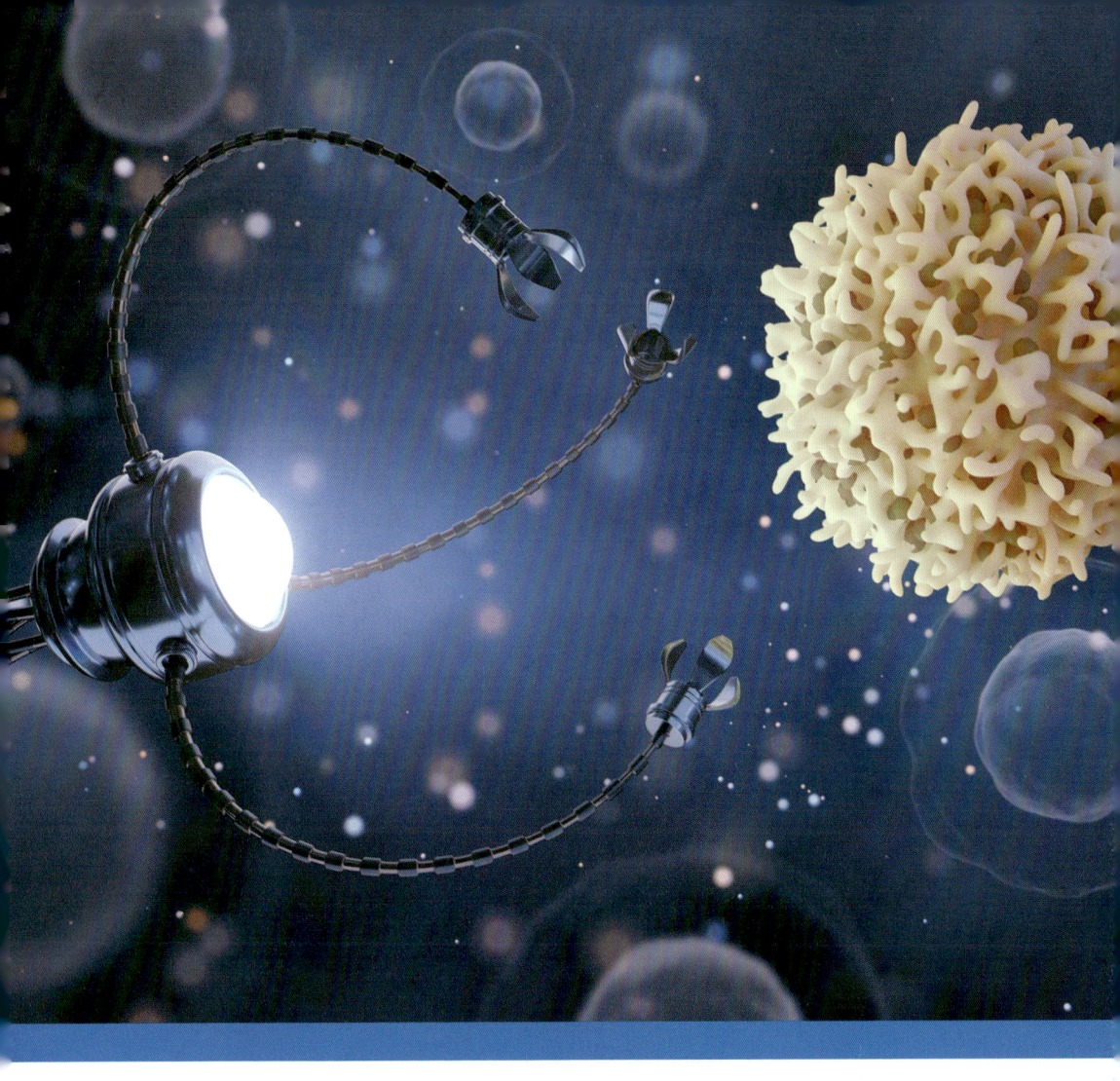

If scientists can figure out the challenges of using tiny robots, these machines may become a promising way to treat patients.

acid. No fuel is needed. Another problem is cost. Micromotors are expensive to make. Cheaper methods must be found.

Only then can micromotors be used in medical treatments.

Eric Diller is a mechanical engineering professor. He works at the University of Toronto. He has developed other types of tiny medical robots. They are less than a millimeter wide. That is less than 0.04 inches. Diller thinks they could be used in surgeries. They will be injected. Then they could be controlled by magnets outside the body. "We could do non-invasive, not just minimally invasive, procedures," Diller says.[8] There would be no cuts. People would heal faster.

ROBOTIC SKIN

Robots can see. Robots can hear. There is even one robot that is an electronic nose. It can smell. Scientists are still working on the sense of touch. Scientists want to build a robotic arm that can be given to people who have lost an arm. It would work like

THE ELECTRONIC NOSE

Scientists at the Monterrey Institute of Technology in Mexico built an electronic nose. The nose senses the chemicals that create smells. It can smell urine, blood, and sweat. It can be mounted on a robotic cart. Then it can track down the smell. Researchers plan to use it for search and rescue missions.

a fully human arm. This requires a sense of touch. Touch tells a person whether something is fragile or soft. They will know whether they need to grip it gently.

People feel the sense of touch with their skin. Scientists are working on robotic skin. This skin must do several things. It must know how hard something is being held. It must know if the force is at an angle. It must be able to tell which finger is gripping an object. It must recognize if the whole finger is being used or just the fingertip. Scientists are developing sensors that can do all of these things. They also need to write the

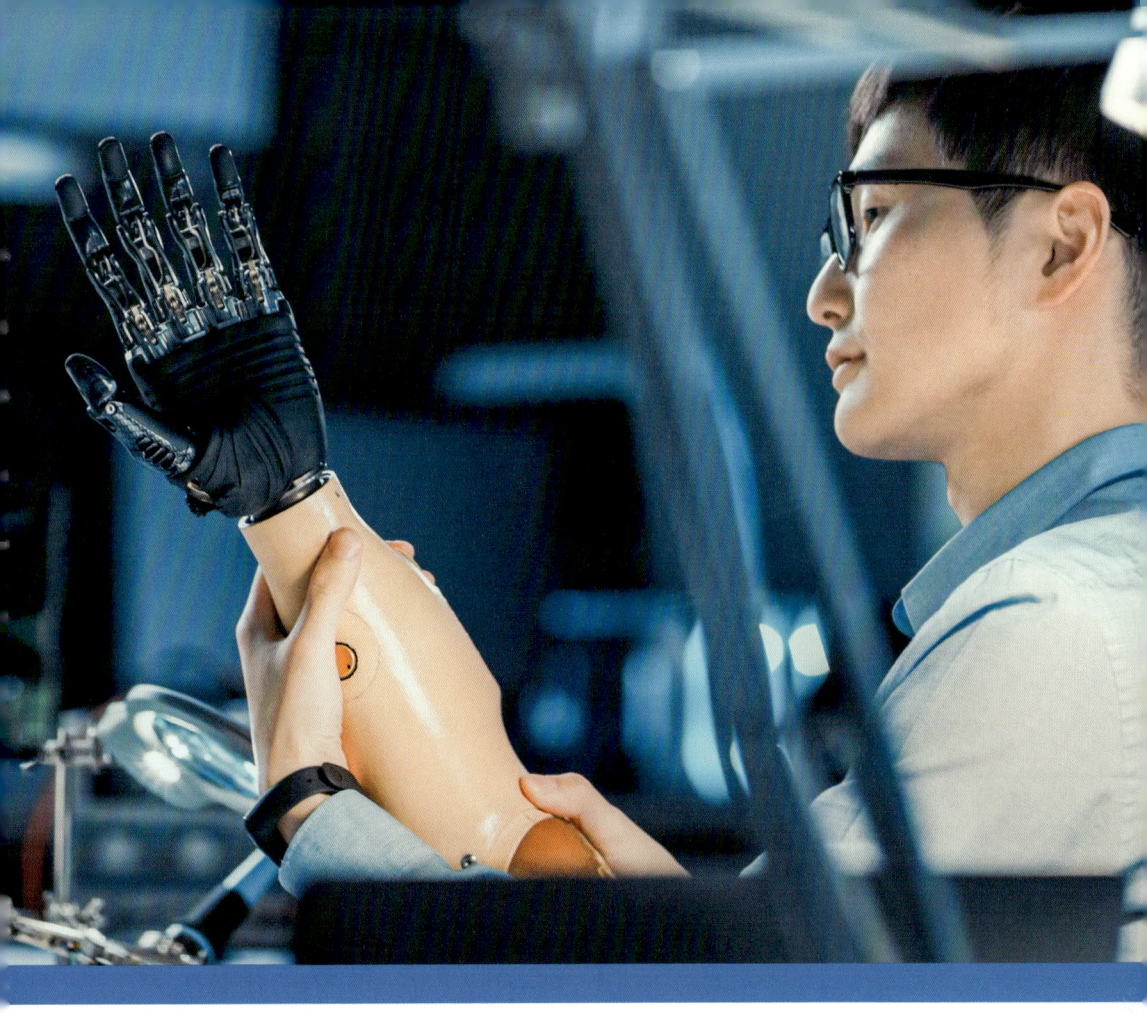

Scientists hope to one day add robotic skin to artificial arms.

computer programs that can respond correctly to the data from these sensors. This can help a person grip an object with the right strength.

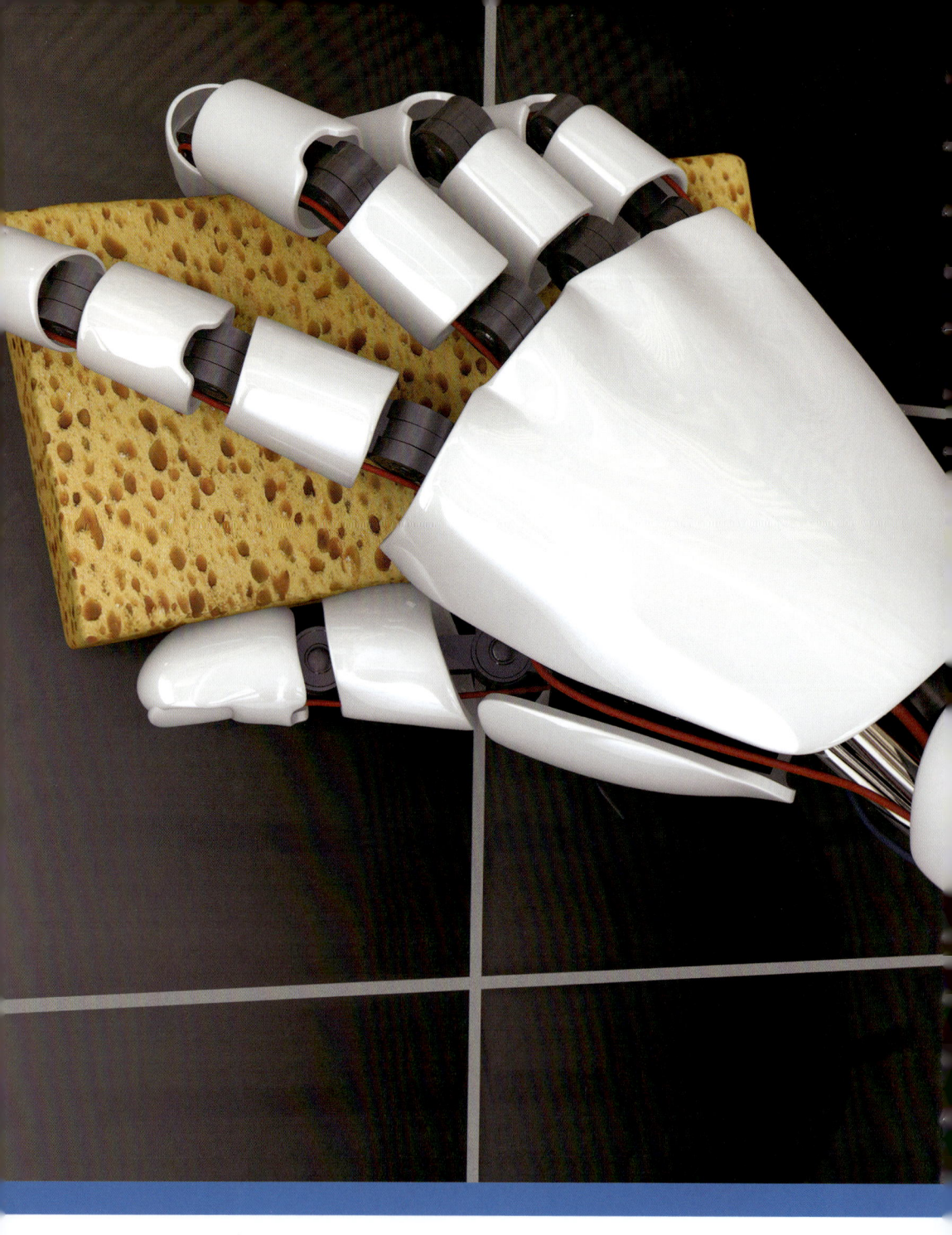

Inventing better robotic hands could make new kinds of robots possible.

Scientists at Harvard University and the Massachusetts Institute of Technology have worked on this. These schools are both in Cambridge, Massachusetts. The scientists made a glove. It has 548 sensors. The sensors are on the glove's fingers and its palm. They signal when the glove touches something. There is one signal for a light touch. There is another for a firm touch. Lifting a light object sends one signal. Lifting a heavy object sends another. "We've always wanted robots to do what humans can do, like doing the dishes or other chores. If you want robots to do these things, they must be able to manipulate objects really well," said Subramanian Sundaram.[9] Sundaram was a graduate student working on the project. A robot or robotic limb needs to have a human sense of touch. Then it can do the things a human does.

A ROBOTIC FUTURE

Students and scientists are working together. They are creating new robots. These robots will be working at new jobs. Many will work in hospitals and clinics.

The next generation of medical robots will improve surgery. They will deliver important

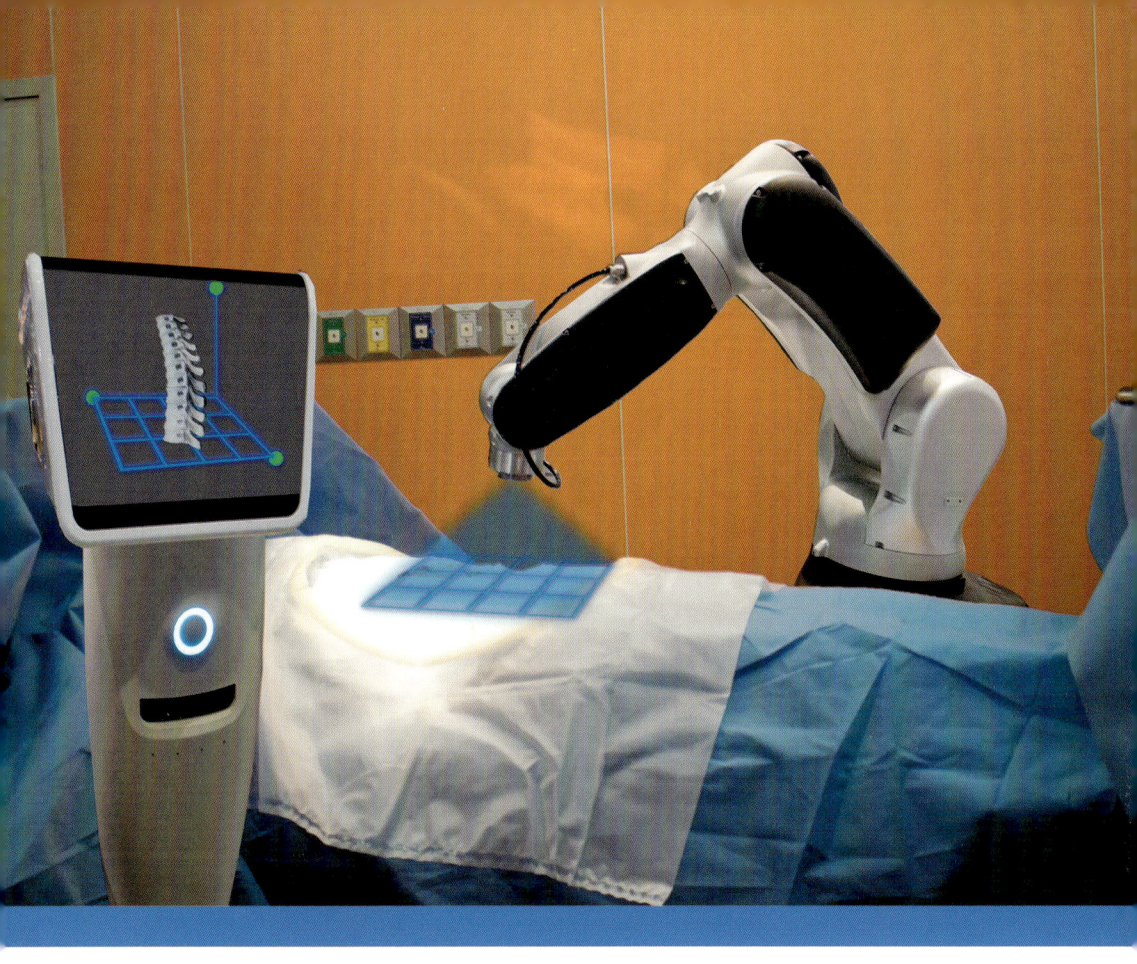

With many scientists at work on medical robots, the future of this technology is bright.

items to patients, nurses, and doctors in hospitals. They will help people heal and recover from injuries and illnesses. Medical robots will continue to make a big difference in the lives of patients across the globe.

GLOSSARY

active

describing a robot able to act on its own

biopsy

a tissue sample that will be tested for disease

CT scan

a picture showing the inside of a patient's body

femur

the upper leg bone

incision

a surgical cut

passive

describing a robot controlled by a person

rehabilitation

exercises or treatments that restore health, also known as rehab

SOURCE NOTES

INTRODUCTION: ROBOTIC SURGERY IN ACTION

1. Quoted in "About Transoral Robotic Surgery," *YouTube: Mount Sinai Health System*, April 12, 2012. www.youtube.com.

CHAPTER ONE: WHAT IS THE HISTORY OF ROBOTICS IN HEALTH CARE?

2. Quoted in Erik Sofge, "The Robotic Doctor Is In," *Popular Mechanics*, March 12, 2013. www.popularmechanics.com.

CHAPTER TWO: HOW DO MEDICAL ROBOTS WORK?

3. "Robotic Surgery: A Facebook Live Discussion with Dr. Bahareh Nejad," *YouTube: UC Davis Health*, December 17, 2019. www.youtube.com.

4. Quoted in "Meet MITRA: The Robot and Its Creators," *YouTube: Analytics India Magazine*, January 4, 2018. www.youtube.com.

CHAPTER THREE: HOW ARE DOCTORS USING ROBOTS TODAY?

5. Quoted in Stacy Weiner, "Robots Make the Rounds," *AAMC*, July 12, 2019. www.aamc.org.

6. Quoted in Weiner, "Robots Make the Rounds."

7. Quoted in Weiner, "Robots Make the Rounds."

CHAPTER FOUR: WHAT'S NEXT FOR ROBOTICS IN HEALTH CARE?

8. Quoted in Edd Gent, "These Tiny Robots Could Be Disease-Fighting Machines Inside the Body," *NBC News*, March 30, 2018. www.nbcnews.com.

9. Quoted in Rob Matheson, "Sensor-Packed Glove Learns Signatures of the Human Grasp," *MIT News*, May 29, 2019. https://news.mit.edu.

FOR FURTHER RESEARCH

BOOKS

Kathryn Hulick, *Robotics and Medicine.* San Diego, CA: ReferencePoint Press, 2018.

Karen Latchana Kenney, *Cutting-Edge Robotics*. Minneapolis, MN: Lerner Publications, 2019.

Cecilia Pinto McCarthy, *Bionics in Health Care*. San Diego, CA: BrightPoint Press, 2022.

INTERNET SOURCES

Lianne Kolirin, "Talking Robots Could Be Used to Combat Loneliness and Boost Mental Health in Care Homes," *CNN*, September 8, 2020. www.cnn.com.

Jason Slotkin, "Meet 'Spot': The Robot That Could Help Doctors Remotely Treat COVID-19 Patients," *NPR*, April 24, 2020. www.npr.org.

Stacy Weiner, "Robots Make the Rounds," *AAMC*, July 12, 2019. www.aamc.org.

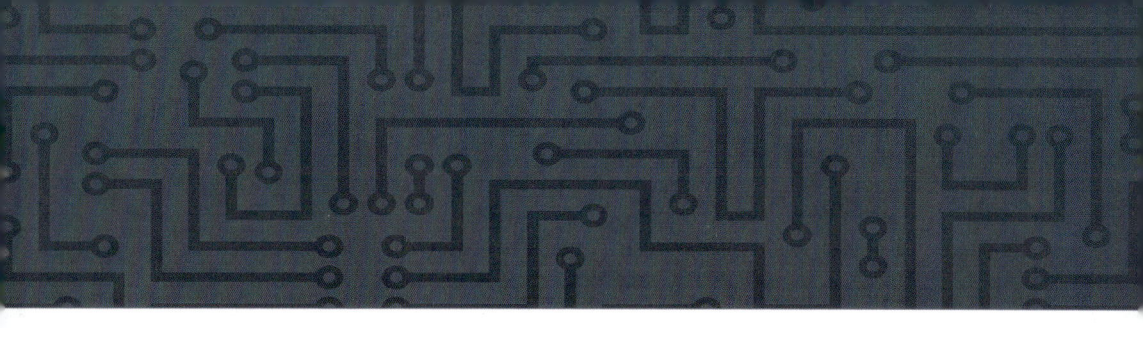

WEBSITES

Aethon: Mobile Robots for Health Care
https://aethon.com/mobile-robots-for-healthcare/

The website of Aethon, the makers of the TUG delivery robot, explores the jobs that the robot does. It also includes videos showing the robot in action.

da Vinci Systems
www.davincisurgery.com

This website from Intuitive, the makers of the da Vinci surgery robot, explains how the robot works and what kinds of surgery it can perform.

Institute of Electrical and Electronics Engineers: What Is a Robot?
https://robots.ieee.org

This website from the Institute of Electrical and Electronics Engineers explores what robots are. It also includes quotes from robot experts about the future of robotics.

INDEX

cleaning robots, 47–49
computers, 10, 14, 24, 28, 34, 69
COVID-19 pandemic, 28, 54, 57
CyberKnife, 41–43

da Vinci surgery system, 21, 40
delivery robots, 24, 29–31, 33, 43–46
Diller, Eric, 66
Dupont, Pierre, 58–60

Genden, Eric M., 11

heart valves, 40, 58–61

laparoscopic surgery, 20–21

micromotors, 62–66
MITRA, 28–29, 30, 36–37, 57
motors, 31–33

NASA, 14–15
Nejad, Bahareh, 35

PROBOT, 18
PUMA 200, 17

rehabilitation, 49–53
Ritz, Jennifer, 47–48
ROBODOC, 18–19
robotic arms, 6, 8–9, 12, 15, 16, 21, 32, 41–42, 67
robotic catheter, 60
robotic skin, 67–68

sensors, 27–30, 60–61, 68–69, 71
Sundaram, Subramanian, 72
surgery robots, 6–9, 14–23, 25–27, 32, 33, 35, 37, 38–41, 58–61, 66, 72

tele-robots, 54–56
toys, 14
Turner, Mary Jane, 45–46

ultraviolet light, 47–48
Unimate, 12

Wagner, Andrew, 22–23

IMAGE CREDITS

Cover: © Monopoly919/Shutterstock Images
5: © Monopoly919/Shutterstock Images
7: © Mad.vertise/Shutterstock Images
8: © Mad.vertise/Shutterstock Images
10: © Denes Farkas/iStockphoto
13: © Gamma-Keystone/Getty Images
17: © Roger Ressmeyer/Corbis Historical/VCG/Getty Images
19: © Terelyuk/Shutterstock Images
21: © thelinke/iStockphoto
22: © Mad.vertise/Shutterstock Images
23: © Red Line Editorial
25: © Chesky_W/iStockphoto
26: © Roman Zaiets/Shutterstock Images
29: © Adnan Abidi/Reuters/Alamy
32: © August Phunitiphat/Shutterstock Images
34: © Monkey Business Images/Shutterstock Images
36: © DorobantuM/Shutterstock Images
39: © Master Video/Shutterstock Images
42: © Hugh Nutt Photography/Alamy
45: © JHVEPhoto/Shutterstock Images
46: © StockSeller_ukr/iStockphoto
49: © natatravel/iStockphoto
51: © Casanowe/iStockphoto
52: © VTT Studio/Shutterstock Images
55: © Zapp2Photo/Shutterstock Images
57: © Dilara Mammadova/Shutterstock Images
59: © pirke/Shutterstock Images
60: © Siwakorn TH/Shutterstock Images
63: © Meletios Verras/iStockphoto
65: © K_E_N/iStockphoto
69: © Gorodenkoff/Shutterstock Images
70: © MakaronProduktion/iStockphoto
73: © Monopoly919/Shutterstock Images

ABOUT THE AUTHOR

Sue Bradford Edwards is a Missouri nonfiction author. She writes about social science, science, and current events. She is the author of twenty-nine books for children, including many about health care.